Home Beauty Clinic

Fully Revised & Updated

Parvesh Handa

Translated by

Dr. Usha Manohar

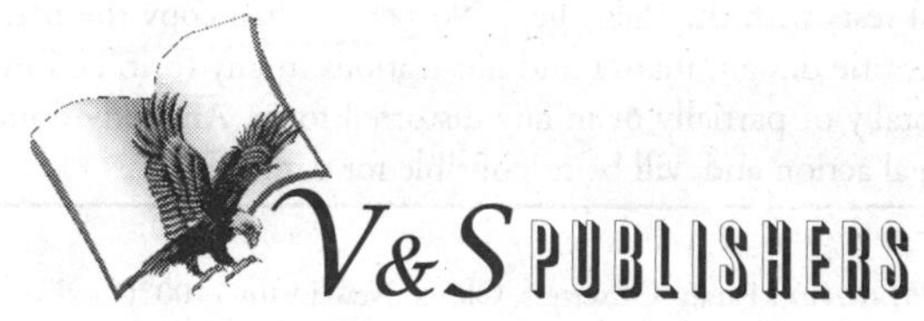

Published by:

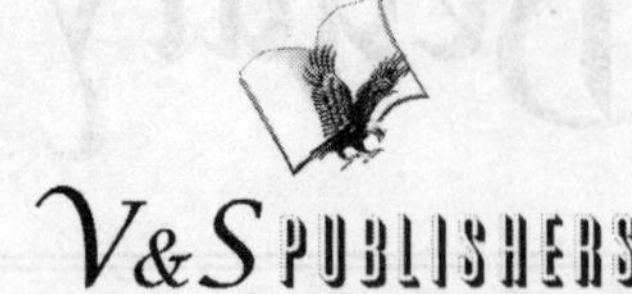

F-2/16, Ansari Road, Daryaganj, New Delhi-110002
☎ 011-23240026, 011-23240027 • *Fax:* 011-23240028
Email: info@vspublishers.com • *Website:* www.vspublishers.com

Branch : Hyderabad
5-1-707/1, Brij Bhawan (Beside Central Bank of India Lane)
Bank Street, Koti, Hyderabad - 500 095
☎ 040-24737290
E-mail: vspublishershyd@gmail.com

ISBN 978-93-813849-6-1

Edition 2013

Printed at : Param Offsetters, Okhla, New Delhi-110020

Home Beauty Clinic

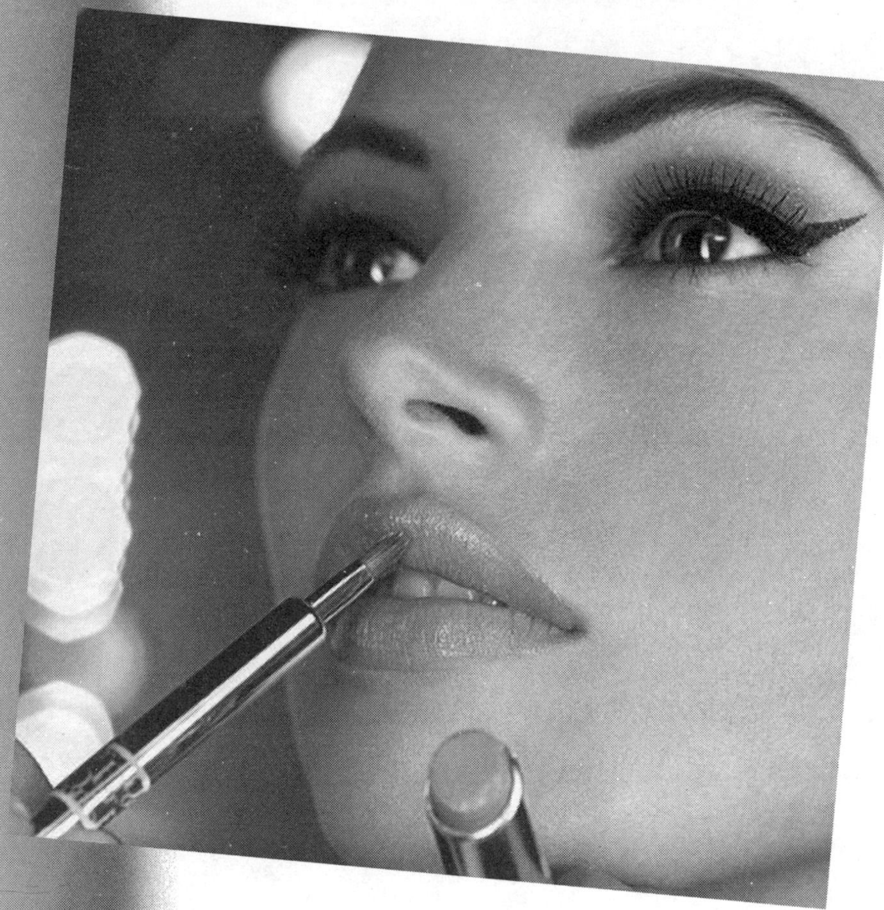

Disclaimer

The information provided in this book is designed to provide helpful information on the subjects discussed. This book is not meant to be used, nor should it be used, to diagnose or treat any medical condition. For diagnosis or treatment of any medical problem, consult your own physician. The publisher and the author are not responsible for any specific health or allergy needs that may require medical supervision and are not liable for any damages or negative consequences from any treatment, action, application or preparation, to any person reading or following the information in this book.

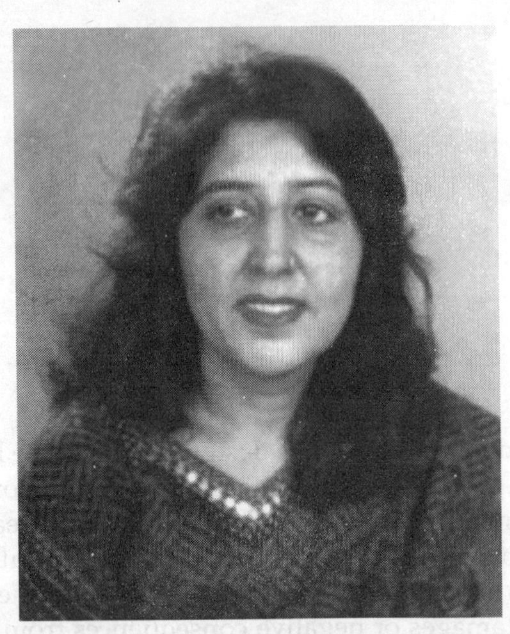

Introducing the Author

Mrs Parvesh Handa is a trained and famous beautician. She is running her clinic for the last many years. She is particularly well-versed in indigenous cosmetics made with herbs and roots. She has done a lot of research in this field. Apart from being a beautician, she is an able writer. More than 500 of her articles on beauty-care have been published in Punjabi, Hindi and English magazines and journals both in India and abroad. She is a regular contributor to the 'beauty columns' in many magazines and newspapers like Nav Bharat Times, Hindustan, Tribune, Indian Express, National Herald, Surya India, Manorama, Griha Shobha, and others.

Publisher's Note

The art of personal beautification by decorative aids is as ancient as human civilization itself. Ever since the universe came into being the female of the species has recognised the importance of her personal charms and the impact of her beauty and physical endowments. Interestingly, however, the concept of beauty, beauty-aids, and clothes and dresses keep on changing with times. In good old days, the yardstick of beauty was restricted to fair complexion, tallish built and large attractive eyes. Today, apart from these concepts, much stress is laid on an attractive and impressive personality, which includes the way of talking, walking, moving in society, choice of clothes and manners in every walk of life.

Formerly, women preferred home made cosmetics and most of them were experts at making their own lotions and creams. However, today, it is the day of the beauticians, and of ready-made cosmetics of various makes. Nevertheless, the aim remains unchanged: To aid woman to look beautiful and attractive and to help her keep herself youthful.

With the expansion of their field of activities, women today have become more aware of personal looks. In this competitive age, it has not only become necessary for every woman to look a class by herself, it has become almost imperative. Although every woman may not have the fairy-tale look of Cindrella or the legendary face of a 'Helen of Troy' who 'launched a thousand ships', there always is something peculiar and charming in every woman, a natural attraction that makes her look bewitching. It is, therefore, necessary for her to enhance that intrinsic charm by hiding her natural deficiencies, if any. And, this is where the art of beautification steps in, coming to their help at the time of need. But, it is not every woman that is acquainted with this art. Beautification does not mean applying creams and powders, it is much more than that.

If your skin is not soft and flawless, if your body is not proportionate or is unhealthy, no amount of cosmetics is going to help you, however costly and effective they may profess to be. Cosmetics will prove futile to enhance your personality. You will have to exert yourself to make the best of the basic elements of beauty you possess. That depends upon your art and your aesthetic sense. A beautician will make you aware of other things, apart from cosmetics, that go into making you look beautiful.

In big cities and metropolises, there is an abundance of beauty-aids, beauty clinics, health clubs and short-term courses. Not so in smaller towns. Moreover, not many women can avail themselves of these facilities. For an average Indian housewife, a visit to a beauty clinic is a luxury to be enjoyed only for marriages or other parties, otherwise she cannot afford these regularly. Where does she turn to, then? Probably, to an authentic book than to unskilled and half-learnt methods picked up at random. It was since long that such an independent book on this subject was in great demand and its absence was badly felt. It was necessary to have a book which could satisfy the various needs of a beauty-conscious woman, such as facial, massage, make-up, pedicure, manicure, hairstyle. This could make the maintenance of their beauty a routine and everyday affair. There is a lot of material and a large number of books on this subject but they are either in foreign languages or have been translated into various Indian languages. Therefore, their contents are not very useful or adaptable under our conditions.

This book is an attempt to remove these two shortcomings and to give original and practical shape to it. Mrs Handa, the author of this book, is too well-known to be introduced. She is not only a trained and experienced beautician but has also earned fame as a good writer. She is well-versed in this subject and has long practical experience. Every attempt has been made to make this book practical and useful for women from all walks of life. All aspects of beauty-aid like facial, massage, make-up, exercises, etc., have been given serially, with illustrations.

The methods of indigenous preparation of cosmetics has been given in detail at the end of this book which has enhanced the utility of this book further more because these home-made cosmetics are not only economical but they are also a safeguard against any side-effect that sometime develops in the ready-made cosmetics.

It is hoped that the book will prove useful and worth preserving.

–Publisher

CONTENTS

PART 1
FACIAL BEAUTY

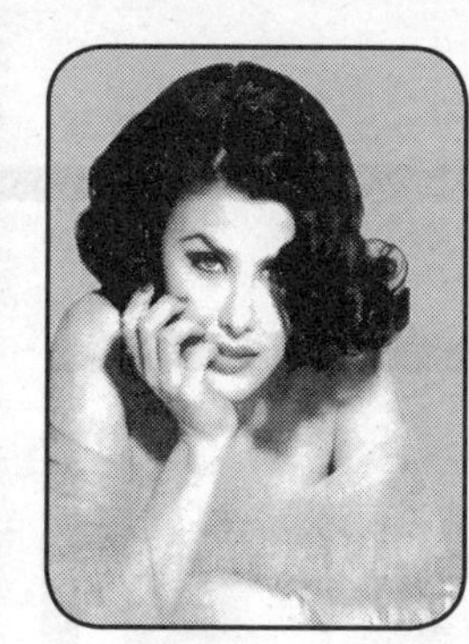

Introduction

PART 2
MAKE-UP

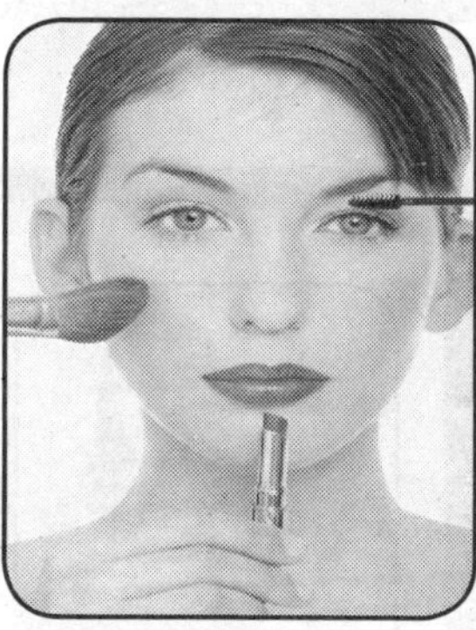

PART 3
CROWNING GLORY

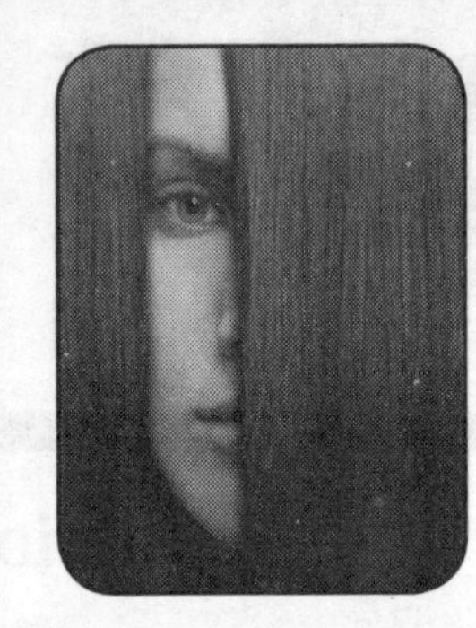

PART 4
BEAUTIFUL BODY

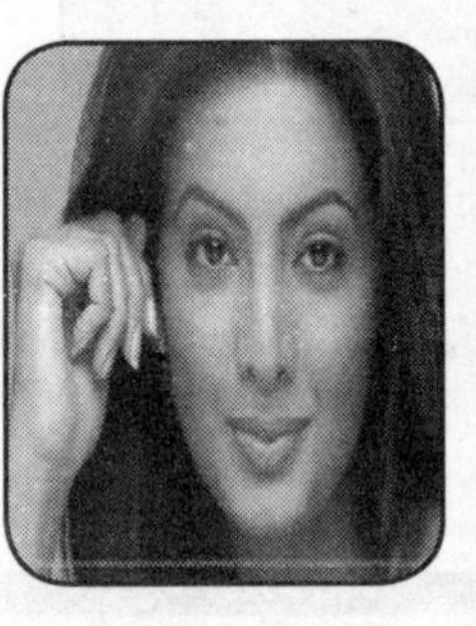

PART 5
HOME-MADE BEAUTY PRODUCTS

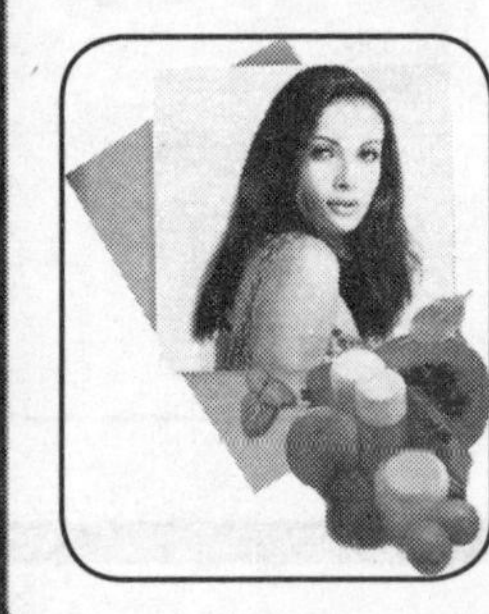

Author's Note

Beautification is no less important today than what it was centuries ago. However, the only difference that has come up is that while the basic concept is the same, the methods have undergone a sea of change. In ancient days, people valued fair complexion, lean waist and attractive eyes. Today, apart from these traditional notions of beauty, much attention is given to personality. A woman today must know the correct use of all beauty-aids so as to make herself attractive and impressive. A flawless posture, correct social manners and exercises play an important part in developing physical beauty. It is, therefore, imperative to acquire a thorough know-how of this art.

During the last two decades the working woman has understood the importance of beautification more than ever before. Sales of beauty-aids and the mushrooming of beauty clinics are the living examples of the above statement. But, the point is how many women have been able to make themselves aware of basic principles of beauty-aids, the importance of figure, good health, soft skin and silken hair. Also, how many women have been able to make correct choice of clothes, cosmetics, and the techniques of make-up? Beauty does not lie only in self-decoration, it is primarily good health, making up of natural deficiency, and enhancement of personality. It has normally been seen that in the absence of correct knowledge of the subject, women have used, at times items which do not suit them, causing damage to their natural beauty.

I have been experiencing the necessity of bringing out such a book as would help women to know the beauty-aids and to educate them in the use of cosmetics. It was also felt necessary that the book in question should cover all aspects of beauty care such as facial, massage, make-up, and the like of it, by putting stress on physical exercises and helping women in sorting out their beauty problems. Today, when the ladies are busy in jobs or even in business, it is essential that their personality is enhanced. A working woman may not have the legendary 'Helen of Troy' look, but she should have a personality that is soft, appealing and dignified. An aesthetic sense will not only enhance her personality, it will lend her self-respect also. With these points in view, I have written this book so as to make it practicable and useful for women of all classes and categories.

How far have I been successful in my attempt is up to you to decide.

We will welcome your queries

–Parvesh Handa

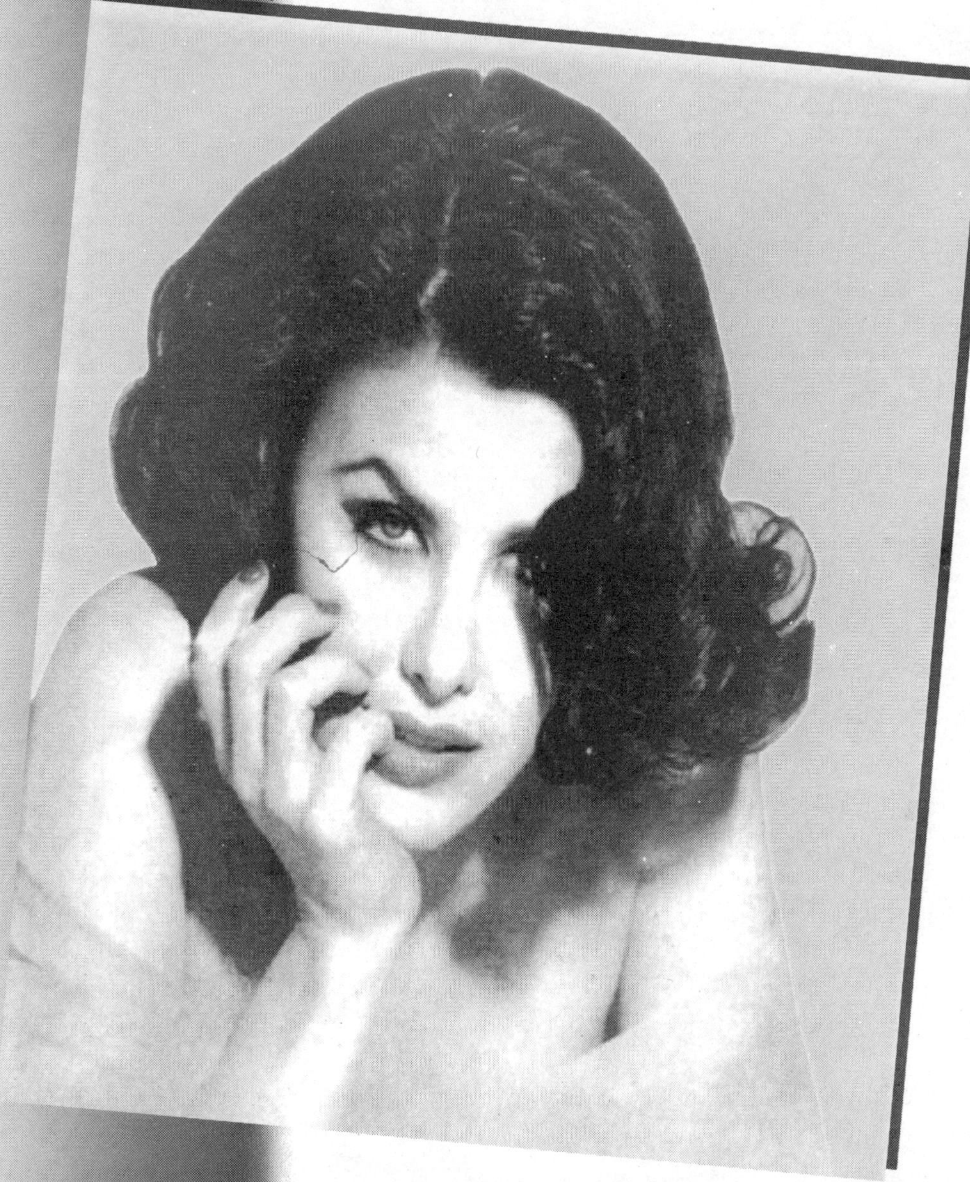

PART 1
FACIAL BEAUTY

WOMEN & BEAUTY FRIENDS FOR LIFE

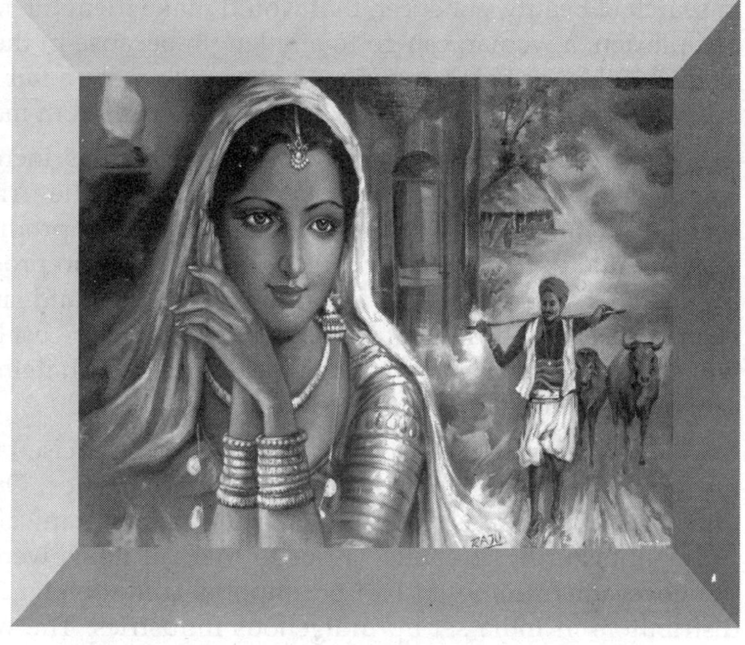

A famous personality once said: "A man is as old as he feels and a woman as old as she looks." And frankly, no woman likes to look old, nor does she relish the idea of looking ordinary. Since the dawn of history, women have diverted their energies towards maintaining their beauty, charm and figures and are still doing today. Poets, with their sensitive vision, have sung paens female beauty in about varied forms. As Kalidas once wrote "A woman's successful decoration is the one which appeals to her dear ones". It cannot be denied that to look plain is not the modern concept. Beautifying oneself and decoration are the best means which women have used to attract men since times immemorial.

Women have employed different methods and measures to heighten their charms down the ages. In ancient India, sixteen methods of self-beautification were practised, which are now popularly known as *solah shringar* in India. These included—filling up the hair-partition with red vermillion; placing a dot (Bindi) on the forehead; kohl or eye-liner in the eyes; turmeric massage followed by a bath; use of perfumed oils; feet coloured red with Alta; henna-dyed palms; a mole on the chin; bedecking with blue lotus; stylizing the hair, use of herbal dyes for the lips like the modern lipstick; nail-polish with lac; sandal-paste massage and profuse use of fragrant herbs and flowers as perfume.

In earlier days beauty-products were not commercially available and women made them at home, displaying their ingenuity and skill. With the passage of time, Indian woman too became conscious of her appearence in the modern sense.

So unquenchable is her thirst for beauty that even a naturally beautiful woman, likes to spend her time and money on beauty-aids or in beauty salon. Despite the rising prices, the rat-race among women seeking cosmetics continues to grow is on demand. The production and sale of cosmetics is on the rise—it is twenty times more than what it was two decades back. In addition to this, there are many women who have a keen interest in home-made beauty-products.

Interestingly, every woman tends to have one beauty complaint or the other. Say, if one woman wants to gain height, the other craves for svelte figure, the third would wish for curly hair and so on. Women seem to be running from pillar to post in search of beauty, enhancer, that would make them the fairest of them all. For a fair complexion, a woman can go to any length because in the Indian society fair skin is always looked as being superior to others. To wear a fair complexion is a dream for every girl because dark skin is considered a curse, from marriage point of view.

The production of toiletries and cosmetics has increased considerably in our country in the last couple of decades especially, with the arrivel of popular international cosmetics brands. Most Indian companies produce products which are comparable with the international market. Till 1961, there was no production-tax on these items. But in 1961, a heavy tax was levied on these items and since then the tax rates have been increasing. The market is also flooded with low-cost but sub-standard cosmetics which contain highly skin-damaging chemicals. Such items, instead of aiding beauty, cause permanent damage to the skin.

According to the statistics available with the excise-tax department, the country has approximately 1200 manufacturers of cosmetics. Out of these only one-third units are running effectively. In 1909, Abraham Patanwala established the first unit for manufacturing cosmetics. Prior to that, all items were imported. In 1954, when the government imposed ban on imports, some foreign companies and their main distributors in India set up indigenous industries. The world renowned Max-Factor Company started its unit in India in 1954. In 1959, the Gala of London started functioning. The Ponds Company set up its factory in Chennai in 1966; Lakme started its production in 1969. Thus, a wide network of companies came into being. Some known names in this field are Johnson & Johnson, J.K. Helen Curtis, Hindustan Lever, Godrej, Colgate-Palmolive, Chambor, Revlon, Garnier, Procter and Gamble, Reveon, Mabellene, et. al.

1. FACIAL SKIN

Do you have a soft, smooth, clear, attractive and glowing skin? If so, you are blessed. But, mind you, the beauty of your skin will not last for ever. With advancing age, there is no guarantee that you will continue to have that fresh youthful look; you will have to exert to keep it as it is. Normally, worries and tensions, coupled with climatic effect, tell upon the skin and many women look aged even in their prime. There are three types of facial skin which are: normal skin, dry, and oily skin.

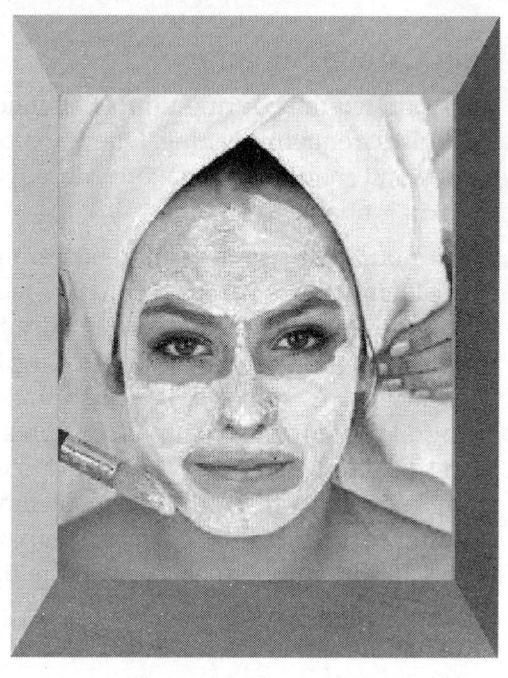

However, there is also a special skin type which is very common these days. It is called Combination Skin. In this skin type the region that covers the forehead, nose and chiw has oily skin. This area is commonly called the 'T' zone. The rest of the face has norma to dry skin.

Normal Skin: This type of skin is one of the best types which retains freshness, attraction and flush for long. It requires very light make-up. Face should be washed with soft water. If normal tap water in your area is hard, soften it by adding a little 'borax powder' to it. In order to retain the glow of your skin, it is imperative to wipe off your make-up before going to bed with a good cleansing cream. Do not use make-up at least once a week so as to let your skin breathe fresh air.

Dry Skin: This type of skin is sensitive to the weather and is prone to wrinkles. Protect it against the wind, Sun and water. Dry skin should not be washed with cold water and facewash, nor should astringent lotions be used. Instead, after cleaning it every night, before bed-time, it is best to use a good moisturizer which can give some freshness to the skin. It should be non-alcoholic, because alcohol dries the skin. The moisturizer should be spread slowly on the face to in an outward motion either with cotton or fingers. Apply the moisturizer on your neck and other parts which are exposed. Diet, which rich in vitamins A, B, C, D should be consumed.

Oily or Greasy Skin: This type of skin is prone to pimples and dark spots. It therefore, requires frequent cleaning, at least thrice a day. Use of sulphur soap is helpful, also, cleaning your face at night with some good quality cleansing milk or with unboiled milk is a good remedy. Avoid greasy food. Your intake of water should be at least six glasses a day. If your skin is allowed to remain greasy, pimples and blackheads appear. A greasy skin does not require make-up. Steaming once a week is an effective method to keep the skin flawless. Use a face-pack after steaming. Face-packs are available in the market but they can also be made at home. The kind of face-pack which would best suit your skin depends on your skin type.

Skin Care in Summer

Your skin requires during utmost attention summer, as sweating makes your skin sticky. It requires frequent cleaning. Due to exposure to the Sun and hot winds, the skin becomes carped and complexion shallow. Moreover, the pores get clogged due to perspiration and the skin is unable to breathe.

If you have a greasy skin, steaming once a week is advisable, if you have a dry skin steam it once a fortnight. For steaming, a special electrical gadget is used. But if you are doing it at home, the procedure is simple – boil water in a pot and place your face on it from a distance so that the rising steam touches your face. Spread a towel on your head to prevent the steam from escaping. 4-5 minutes of steaming is sufficient. After this, sprinkle your face with ice-cold water so as to close the open pores. Regular steaming keeps the skin glowing.

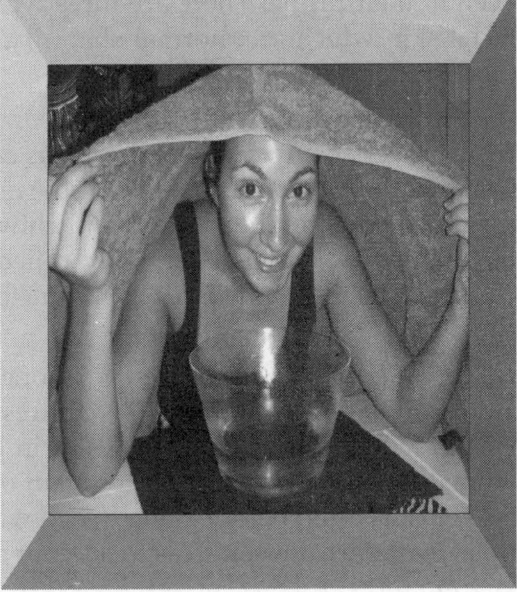

Quick hints to help protect your skin during summer:

- Use facewash at least once in a day.
- Clean your face and neck with a good cleansing-milk.
- Use a good astringent for oily skin.
- After cleaning your face, take an ice cube and massage it all over your face in slow motion.
- Wash your face with cold water at least thrice a day.
- A light massage, with a night cream, before going to bed is useful, but the quantity of cream should be small because in summer you don't want to be all greasy.

Skin Care in Winter

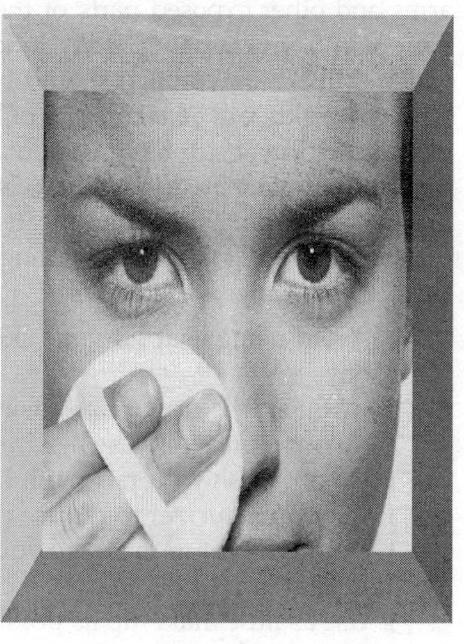

The icy winter winds greatly damage your skin and with it comes skin chapping which is a common problem. But, the skin type which is most vulnerable to cold is dry skin which cracks easily if remains uncared for. Many-a-time cracked skin bleeds too. It is, therefore, necessary to avoid long exposures. Also you have to take care of the other exposed parts of your body such as palms, feet, back and neck, etc. Icy winds also dull the complexion of your skin. If the skin is dry, then minimise the use of soap and use a good facewash. Cold cream and olive oil are effective in reducing dryness. But, it is essential to deep-cleanse your face. For deep-cleansing, take a cotton swab, dip it in water and squeeze it. Apply cleansing–milk and gently rub it on your face and neck. Do not use unheated milk as it can lead to opening up of pores on the face. Tomato and raspberry juice best suited for facial cleaning. At night, do not use water after cleansing, instead use a wet towel for wiping. The towel should be dipped in hot water and then squeezed. After this, a facial massage with a skin-tonic mixed with almond oil is beneficial. Massage the skin for at least 10 minutes so as to enable the cream to penetrate the skin.

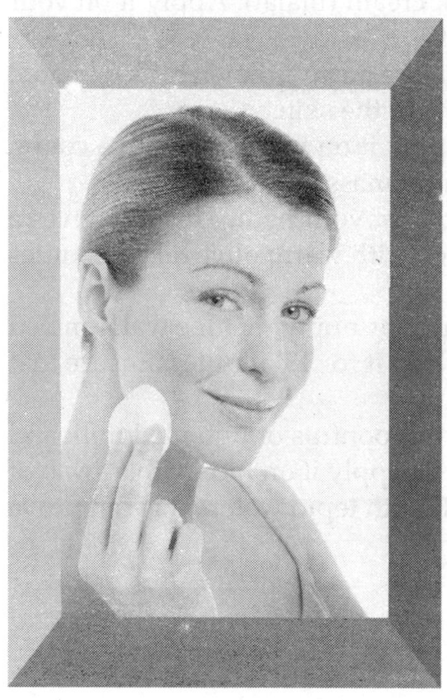

Skin-tonic can be either bought from the market or prepared at home. For home-made tonic—take 50 gms. of marigold petals, soak them in a half a litre of water in a stainless steel pot and warm it on heater. Keep the flame slow. Keep the lid on the pot so that the steam does not escape. Now take pure wax, melt it and mix it with the mixture and heat it on a medium flame for half an hour. When the cream gets cold, fill it in a bottle. This is your skin-tonic. Cold cream is used primarily in winter. For home-made cold creams—peel a cucumber and cut it into small pieces. Take 4 parts of almond oil, 1 part pure wax and put it on low heat. When the two mix completely then add pieces of cucumber and heat on a low flame for 45 minutes. The cucumber pieces should be ¼th of the mixture. Stir slowly while heating. You may add a little perfume for fragrance.

During winter, dry skin will regain its glow only by massaging. Massage your hands, arms and other exposed parts of the body with a good body lotion. This will prevent your skin from chapping. Body lotion can be prepared by mixing lemon juice in rose water. 'Milk cream' (malai) should be applied on wrists and fingers to keep them soft. Dryness of skin can be taken care of by massaging with olive oil, mustard oil or almond oil, followed by a sun bath. A little after sun bath, bathe, with luke-warm water which helps in removing tiredness; and it also increases blood circulation in the veins. To prevent lips from chapping, a light application of cold cream or vaseline on the lips is essential, especially before going to bed. Using chapstick also helps. Some measures to protect the skin during winter is as follows:

- ❒ Avoid using soap. If your skin is oily, wash your face with a facewash twice a day.
- ❒ If you skin is dry use cleansing cream.
- ❒ If your skin is oily use a skin-tonic.
- ❒ Do not wash your face with hot water.
- ❒ Use a moisturizer to reduce dryness of skin.
- ❒ Do not forget to massage your face with cold cream or skin-tonic before going to bed.
- ❒ Use as little make-up as possible if you have pimples.
- ❒ Dry, cold winds often chap the skin. To guard against it, make a paste by adding maida to milk and rubbing it well on the face. Dirt and dust will be removed with the paste leaving the skin soft.
- ❒ If you have a dry and rough skin, take the seeds of watermelon, pumpkin, cucumber and kharbuja (known as charon-magaz) in equal quantities, grind them in milk. Make a paste adding fresh milk cream (malai). Apply it on your face. Leave it for one hour and then wash it off.
- ❒ Take mustard seeds. Clean and grind them. Make a paste either in milk or water. Daily use of this paste is good and adds a glow to the skin.
- ❒ Mix water and vinegar in equal quantities. Apply it on your face with a cotton swab. If the skin is dry, use cold cream for a light massage.
- ❒ Add a spoonful of olive oil to a bucket of water for your bath. This also gives a glow to the skin. If the skin is very dry, massage with warm olive oil 15 minutes prior to your bath.
- ❒ During summer, protect yourself from hot winds by applying lime water mixed with *alsi* oil in equal quantities on your face. Keep it for 15 minutes. Ensure that it does not go into your eyes.
- ❒ For dry skin, take a spoonful of almond oil, 10 spoonfuls of unboiled milk and a pinch of sugar. Mix and beat the mixture well. Apply it on face with a swab of cotton. Let it remain for 15 minutes. Wash it off with tepid water. This can prove to be very useful.

***

2. FACIALS FOR YOU

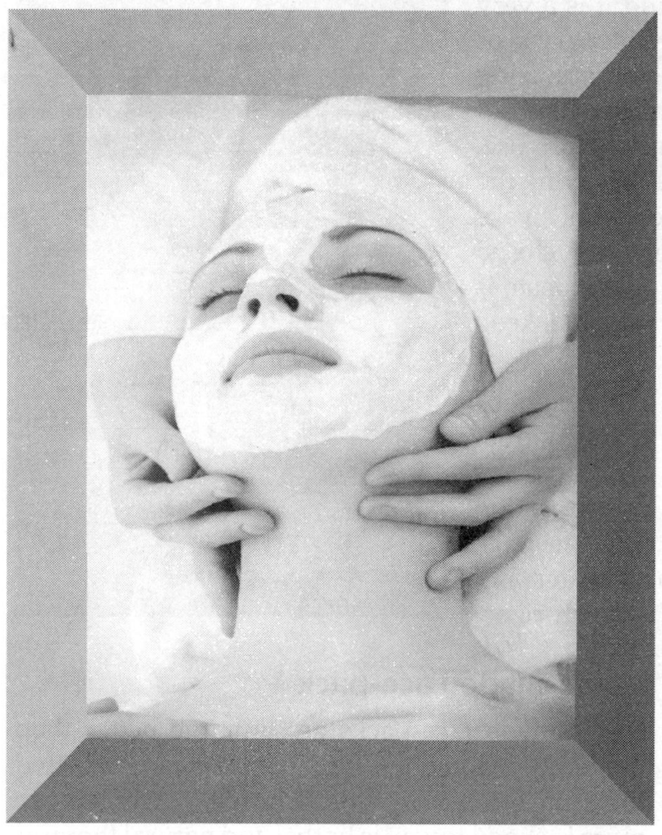

Natural beauty is a blessing but most women tend to lose it by their own negligence, in their bid to outdo each other in modernity. As soon as a girl reaches her adolescence, she gets attracted towards cosmetics which prove harmful for her skin. Excessive use of make-up makes one lose her natural beauty. The pores of the skin clog because of make-up. Clogging prevents carbon dioxide inside our body to exit and fresh oxygen to enter the body. This results in the skin losing its original glow. It becomes very difficult to regain the lost beauty. Facial, once a week, keeps the face attractive. For a facial the face is first thoroughly cleaned. After that it is massaged with a massage cream and steamed. A face-pack is then applied.

Cleaning: Facial is done only on a clean skin. Use a scrubber or cleansing-milk to clean the face. If your skin is oily, wash it with a facewash and tepid water. If the skin is dry, wipe cream with cotton swabs.

Massage: Now your face is ready for a massage. Always keep in mind the nature of your skin while choosing the kind of cream for massage. If your skin is normal or oily then you can use normal cream or an all-purpose cream. If, on the other hand, your skin is dry then use a vitamin based cream. Massage with light pressure of your fingers. Bear in mind that the massage is done with upward strokes. From the inner side to outer side, and from lower to upper parts. (The process of massaging is explained in detail in the next chapter.) The skin around the eyes is extremely sensitive, therefore, the cream should be applied there without any pressure. Massage should be done for about 10-15 minutes so as to get sufficient time for the cream to penetrate the skin. The surplus cream on the face should be wiped off with cotton wool swab.

Steaming: Steaming helps the pores, to open and the skin gets the full benefit of face-pack. Take a pot and boil water in it. Cover your face with a big towel and put it on the mouth of the vessel. You can put peppermint, rose-petals, mint-petals or petals of marigold in the water, if you so desire. Dry your face by patting it gently.

Face-pack: The last step in to open the facial process is applying the face-pack and it is a very important part. You can either buy face-pack or you can also prepare it at home. If you are using a ready-made product, then you must read all the instructions on the label carefully before use. Apply the paste on your face and neck leaving the portion below your eyes. Place cotton wool swabs dipped in rose water or cucumber your closed eyes and lie down calmly. As long as the paste is on your face do not smile or talk. If possible, keep your feet at a higher level.

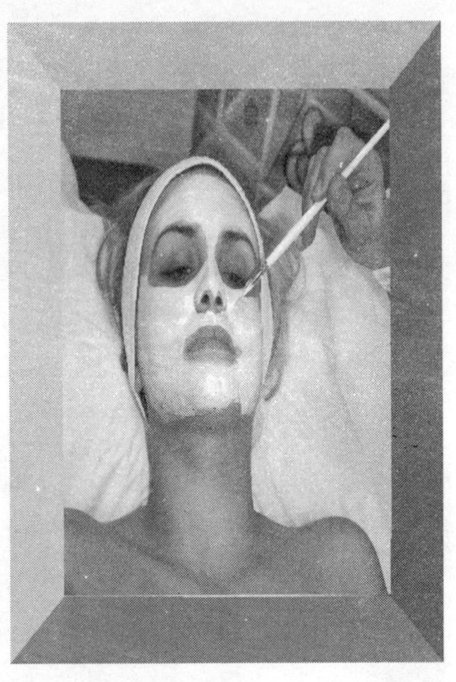

How long should one keep the face-pack on? That varies from individual to individual depending on the nature of the skin and the quality of face-pack. Normally, the duration should be for about 10-20 minutes. Once the pack dries, wash the face with luke-warm water and apply a thin layer of cold-cream or a moisturizer.

Home-made Face-pack

Home-made face-packs are anytime better than the ready-made ones. Indian women are attracted towards make-up, while European women are more inclined towards herbal and natural therapy. Make-up can temporarily enhance your beauty but in the long run, repeated use leaves scars spots and the mature aged look. Home-made face-packs provide natural oil and moisture to the skin. If you look carefully you will find many ingredients in the face-pack in your kitchen. A few quick ways to prepare face-packs at home are as follows:

Egg Pack: Take the yolk of one egg, mix in it 2 spoonfuls of rose water and 1 spoonful of honey and preserve. Use it once a week. It is useful in

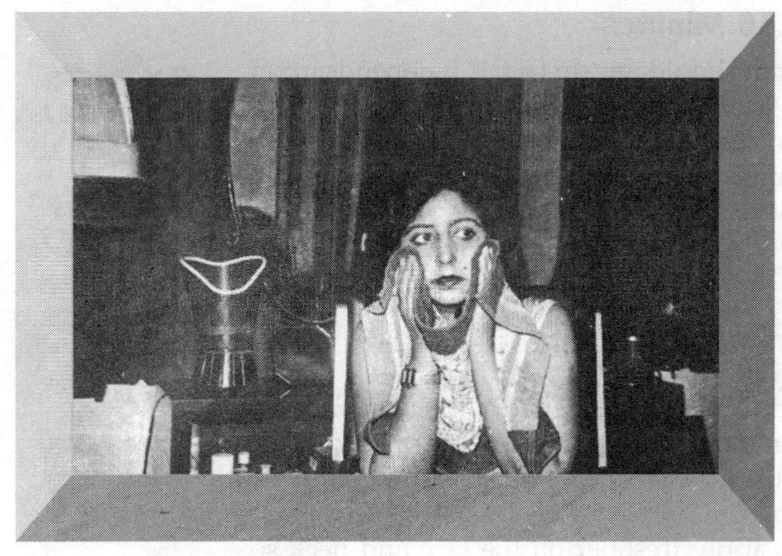

winters. If you have wrinkles, take the white of an egg, beat it, mix in it 3 spoonfuls of oat-powder, 1 spoonful of honey and apply on the face. For very dry skin take the yolk of 1 egg, 2 spoonfuls of orange juice, half a spoon of lemon juice and a few drops of sweet almond oil. Mix it well, beat it and apply it. Keep it on for half an hour before washing it off.

Soyabeans or Masoor Dal (Lentil) Pack: Take 50 grams soyabeans (or masoor dal), soak it in water over-night. Grind it well the next morning into a paste after removing the shells. Mix unboiled milk and almond oil in the paste and apply.

Besan (Gram Flour) Pack: Take 1 spoonful of besan, a pinch of turmeric (haldi), half a spoon of honey and half a spoon of olive oil. Mix it well and apply.

Multani Mud Pack: Take a spoonful of finely ground multani mud, a spoonful of rose water or cleansing-milk and prepare a thick paste. Apply a thick coat on the oily part of your face and a light coat on the dry part. Let it remain for 10 minutes before washing it off with lukewarm water.

Urad Dal Pack: Grind urad dal into a fine powder, mix rose water, glycerine and almond oil, make a paste and apply.

Sandalwood Pack: Make a chandan paste, add rose water and apply it on your face. It has a cooling effect. If the skin is oily, add a small quantity of sulphur to it.

Mint Pack: Grind fresh green mint and apply the paste on your face for 20-25 minutes. It absorbs internal heat from the skin.

Curd Pack: Take 1 spoonful of besan, 2 spoonfuls of curd. Mix well, apply it for half an hour. It is soothing for the skin affected by heat-wave.

Butter coating: If your face is dry due to heat, beat a spoonful of butter in water and apply.

Cucumber Pack: Peel a cucumber and grind it fine. Put unboiled milk in it and apply. It helps to soften the skin.

Home-facial in Quick 30 Minutes

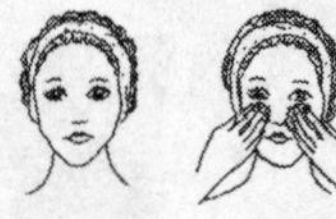
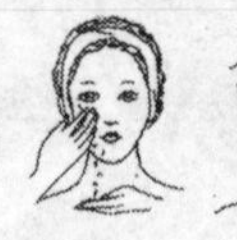
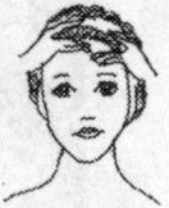
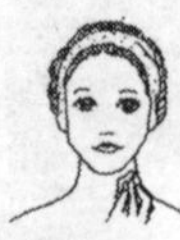
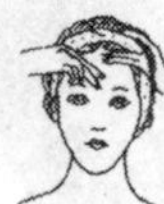
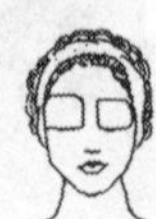
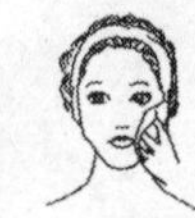

How many times in a month should one do facial? It depends upon your age and the nature of skin. For those who are in the age-group of 14-25 and who have normal skin or at least do not have a very dry skin, facial once a month is sufficient but for those who have dry or dull skin, facial twice a month is necessary. For those who are older, facial once a week is a must so that age does not show on the face.

Ways to do a quick 30 minutes facial:

1. Tie your hair tightly at the back.
2. Clean the face with a cleanser so that make-up and dust particles, if any, are removed. Use a tissue-paper or a facewash and water to clean the face. It is necessary to clean your neck also along with face.
3. Use cotton wool to apply freshner on the face and neck so that the last traces of cleanser are removed.
4. Put moisturizer in dots on your temples, cheeks and chin and then let the skin absorb it.
5. Now wash the face with clean tepid water.
6. Make the face-pack according to the nature of your skin, and apply it on your face and throat, leaving the area around the eyes untouched. Soak the cotton wool in rose water and place it on your eyes. You can use unboiled milk or alcohol-free freshner also, instead of rose water.
7. Now lie down and allow the face-pack to dry for about 20 minutes.
8. Wash away the face-pack. Dry your face and neck by patting with a soft towel and apply a good moisturizer.

3. WRINKLES

With age, wrinkles appear on the face which prematurely give an older look to a young person. For women, in particular, wrinkles are a curse. But, this tendency and the resultant ageing can be checked sufficiently if care is taken when you are still young. Just as balanced diet and regular exercise is important to control the fattening tendency, likewise regular massage of the face is effective to prevent appearance wrinkles and to give the face a fresh look.

Facial massage is an effective way to counter wrinkles. Massage is a slow process and results show only when it is continued for a longer period. It is, indeed, not a magic wand to bring a change overnight. One has to be patient with it. There is, however, no doubt that massage reduces the unattractive fleshiness, tightens the tissues and muscles and increases blood circulation.

Massage is effective if the skin is clean. After having cleaned the face, press it with light but firm pressure while applying a good cream. Trained fingers can hold the skin dexterously and apply unifarm pressure. With passage of time, all visible blemishes like wrinkles, flabbiness, and dead cells vanish and a fresh and young look is restored.

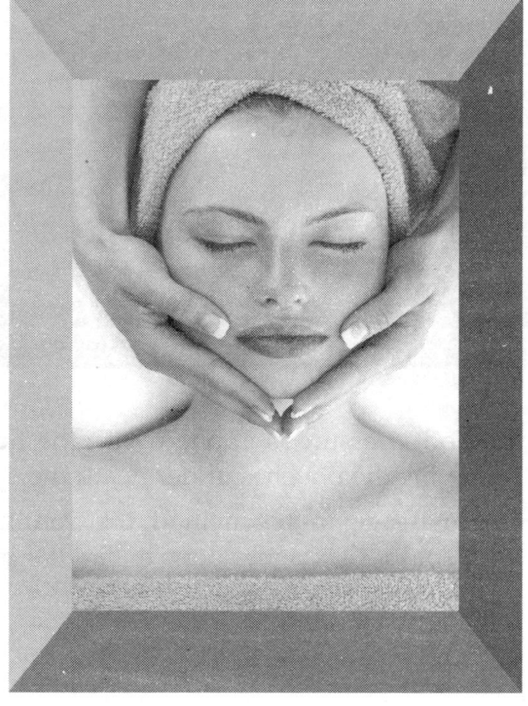

Massage should start from the neck upwards and end at the forehead or temples (see illustration) because there is blood circulation in all veins and tissues by this process. The skin around the eyes is delicate. So it is advisable to apply cream on this part without pressing it. Cream takes 15-20 minutes to get absorbed, so massage for that long. Wipe off extra cream with a cotton wool swab soaked in water.

To protect your hair, tie a cloth or scarf on your head before the massage (see illustration). Hands should be washed with soap. Remove all traces of make-up, otherwise the pores in the skin will be blocked by particles potent in the make-up. If there are blackheads, they should also be removed. If the skin is oily, remove its oiliness either by applying cleansing-milk or PH acid. Fresh lemon juice is also effective in removing oil. A lemon, sliced into half, can be rubbed on the face. If the skin is dry, use a good moisturizer before the massage. If the skin is damp, it is advisable to use some astringent lotion. The best time for massage is before going to bed. Vitamin 'C' cream should be applied before massage, but the quantity of cream should be enough only to give sufficient greasiness to the skin so that the hands and fingers move smoothly on the face. If the face is fleshy and fat, use slimming cream instead of Vitamin 'C' cream.

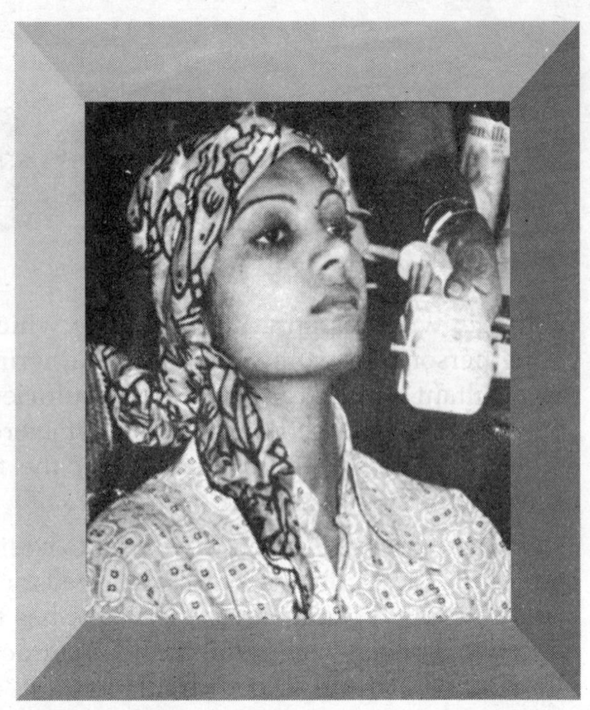

There are many methods of face-massage which are given as follows:

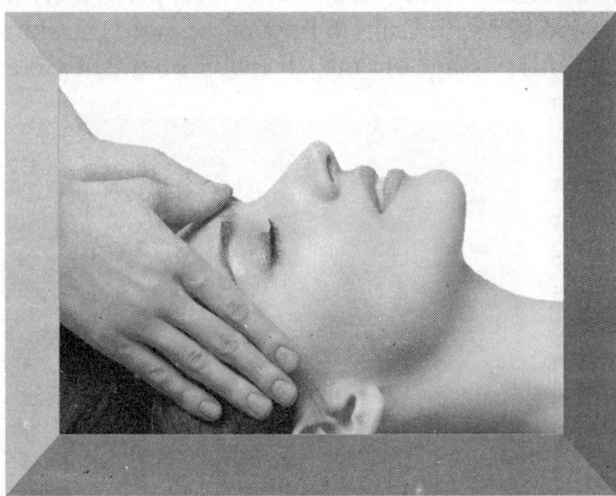

Slow massage: This kind of a massage is done slowly by hitting and vibrating the skin. The skin is pressed lightly with the soft fleshy tips of the fingers. The process starts in a slow speed from the neck, the speed increases as it moves upwards (see illustration). Stroking gives rest to the nerves. Vibration is useful in subduing the pain that caused by massaging. Vibration is produced either by fingers or by an electric gadget, which is called an 'eyebrow massager'.

Massage by pressure: In this method, pressure is applied with the fleshy tips of the fingers. This is effective for removing the pouches under neath the eyes.

Fast massage: In this method, the front half of both the palms is used to massage but with speed. Massage is done in circular motions upwards. It is a quick way to remove wrinkles.

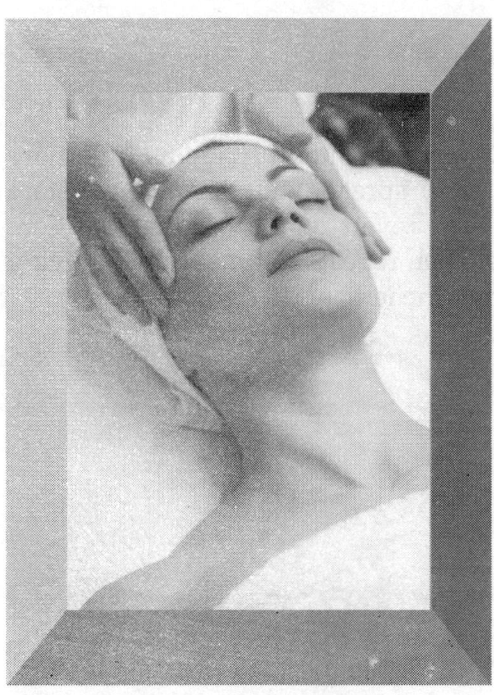

Massage by stroking: In this method, chubby cheeks are stroked with the tip of fingers. If the nose is broad, this method is used (strokes are applied) to both sides of the cheeks, from nose to the temples.

Massage by pinching: In this method, the skin is held, as in pincers, between the thumb and fingers. It is effective for double chin and wrinkles around the jaw.

Massage by kneading: In this method, hands are folded in a fist and the face is pressed as in kneading the flour. The movement is from the chin to cheeks and upwards. This method is very effective for wrinkles.

Facial Exercises

'Face is the index of mind', goes a wise old saying. More so, face is the most attractive part of your personality. Therefore, you should keep your face healthy, soft and young. Facial exercises are useful for a healthy look. These exercises should be done regularly by standing in front of a mirror (in the privacy of your room or bathroom). Some effective exercises are as follows:

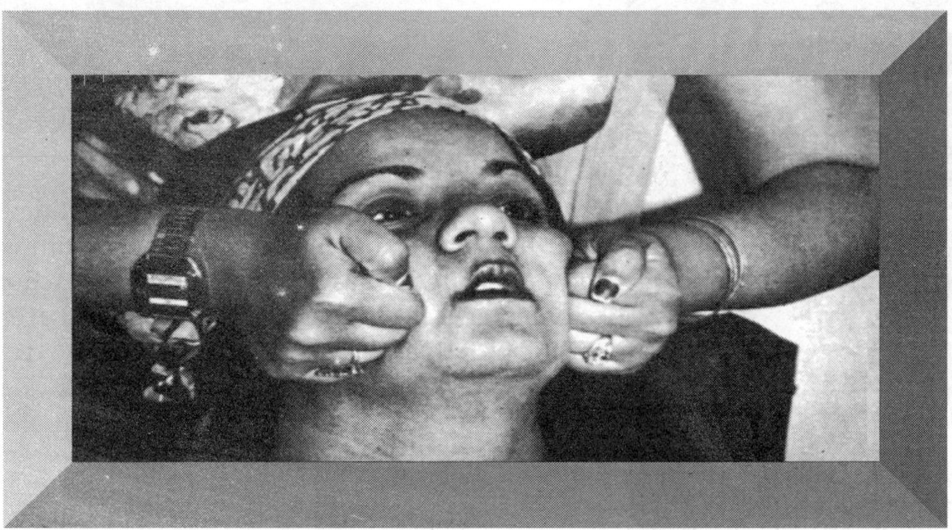

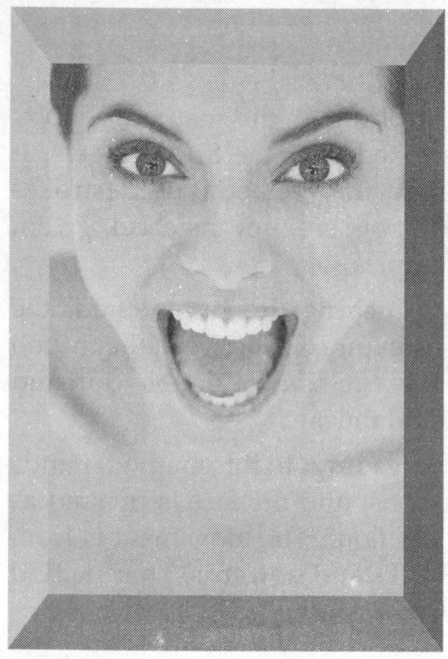

Exercise 1: Open your mouth wide as if you are ready to scream, spread wide your eyes, stare ahead; and then revert to the original position. Do it 5 times. Then repeat it 5 times while moving your head from the left and to right.

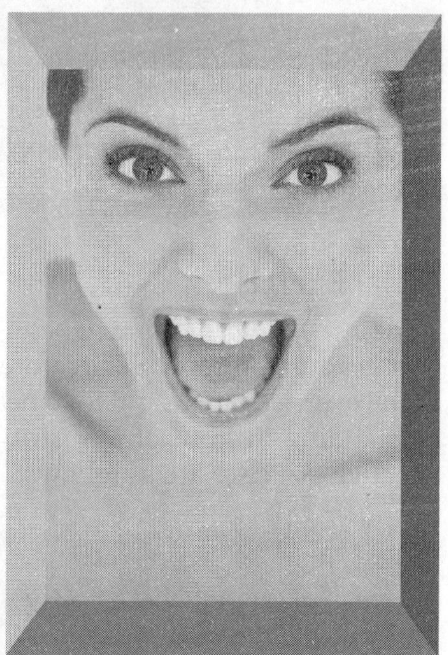

Exercise 2: Press your forehead (near the hair-line) with your fingers and rub it in a backward motion. Lines on the forehead, if any, will disappear by smooth rubbing.

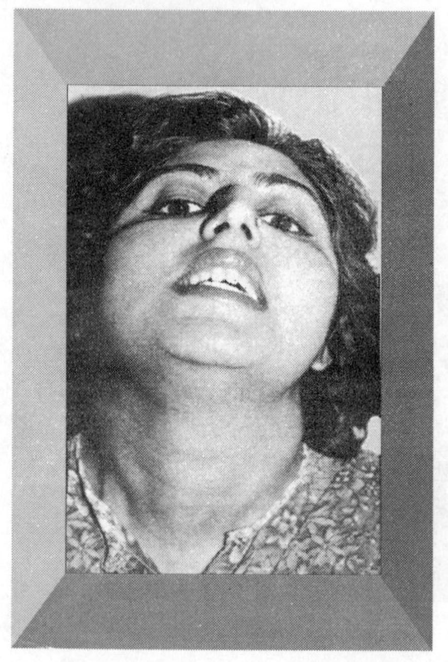

Exercise 3: Open your mouth wide and slide back your head. Now, open and close your mouth while moving your jaw as if munching. This action of opening and closing your mouth is a good exercise for the mouth and jaw. Do it ten times.

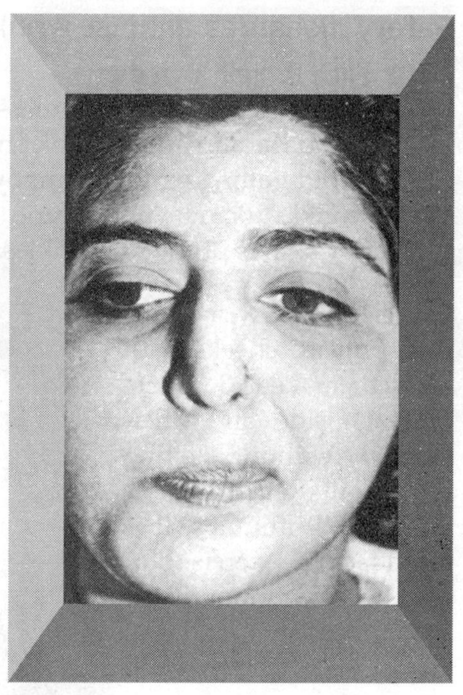

Exercise 4: Sit in front of a mirror. Twist your lips inward. Puff your mouth with air inside it. Now, let there be a laugh on one half of your face once, and on the other half next. Do it 10 times in all. It will smooth your cheeks.

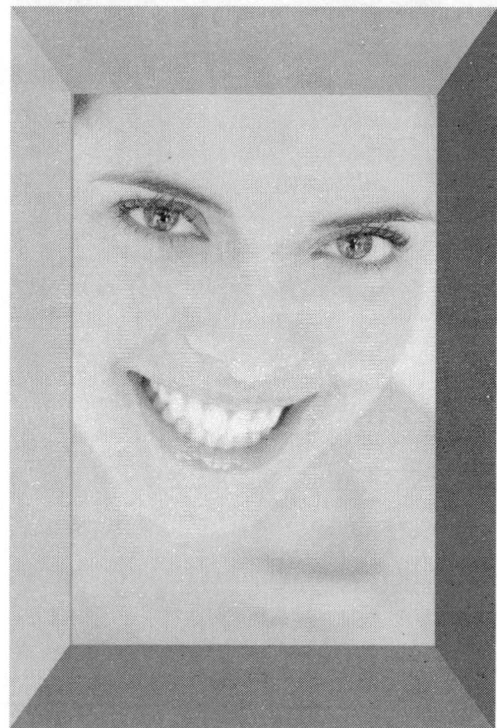

Exercise 5: Keep your face straight in front of a mirror. Press your teeth and spread your lips. Count 10 and revert to normal pose. Do it 10 times.

Safety measures against wrinkles

- ❒ Eat a Protein-rich diet
- ❒ Do regular upward face-massage
- ❒ Avoid the sun and intake of hot things.
- ❒ Avoid getting irritated, annoyed or angry because they quicken development of wrinkles. Be calm and serene, and let your face be peaceful.
- ❒ Dry skin is prone to wrinkles. Regular use of moisturizer is advisable.

Exercise 6: Twist your lips, puff up cheeks with air in them, keep 3 fingers on each side and press slowly, without letting the air out. Remain in this pose for 10 minutes. It is an effective exercise for the cheeks and mouth.

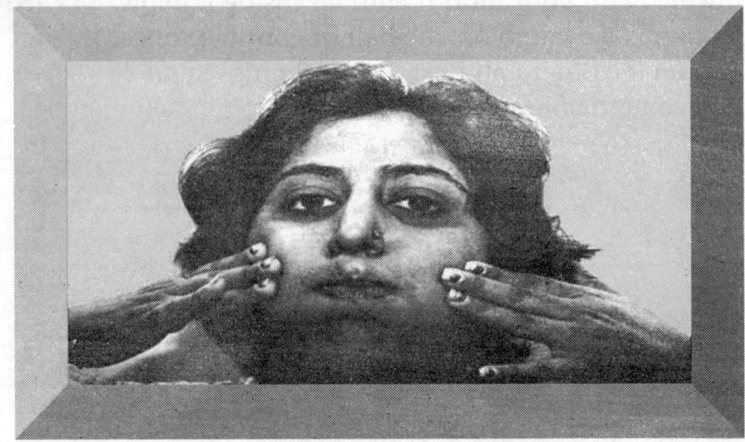

***

4. MARKS AND SPOTS

Any kind of spot or spots on the face spoil the charm of a woman. Every beauty-conscious woman wants to prevent such beauty-deterrents. Spots are of various kinds such as dark spots underneath the eyes, white patches, and small-pox spots. The dark rings below the eyes make a woman look older than her age. Today, about 90 per cent women suffer from tensions which have a massive affect on the skin and eyes. The eyes keep sinking each day and get surrounded by dark circles. Wrinkles also appear around them. This blackishness and wrinkles are not confined to eyes only but spread over the entire face making a person look old for her age.

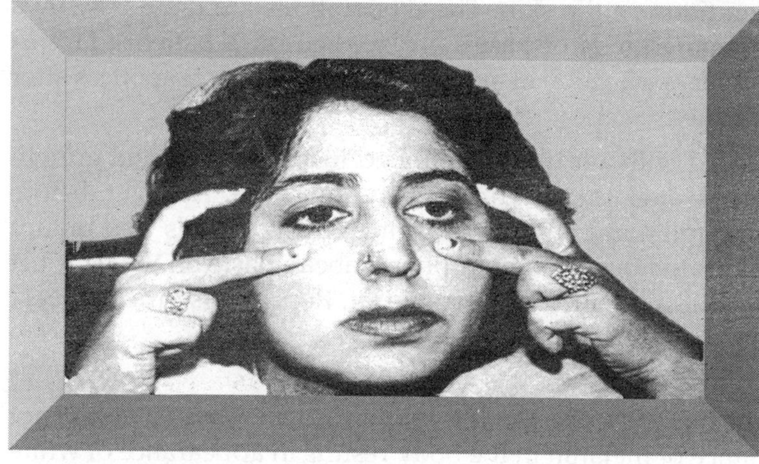

Now you may question as to why these dark spots and wrinkles appear first around the eyes only? The reason is that the skin around eyes is very sensitive and contains a very thin layer of fat. If this fat remains healthy then the eyes do not sink. When the fat gets reduced and becomes dead there is little or no flow of blood in them and the veins cannot hold the eyes at the initial level.

Although, make-up helps in hiding these flaws to a certain extent, it is necessary to control the psychological factors, so as to cure them permanently. Avoid tensions, increase the intake of vitamin 'C', and consult your physician to check for internal disorders, if any. Green vegetables, lemon and orange are very rich in vitamin 'C', which purify blood-carrying veins in the body and maintain the natural glow of the skin. Women should apply only that much make-up which looks natural. It is necessary to clean every trace of make-up at bed time otherwise the pores of the skin get blocked and their activity stops. Thus body-waste remain inside and their rotting process makes the skin unattractive.

Do not rub the area around the eyes, because rubbing may result in shrinking of the skin. Use the middle finger of your left hand and tap lightly. The skin around the eyes remain healthy by applying a mixture of rose water and cucumber juice in that area. You may use anti-wrinkle cream in case of wrinkles or dark spots around your eyes. Quick home-made remedy for this is as follows:

Boil tea-leaves and strain, foment the area below the eyes with this warm decoction.

A light massage by applying almond oil on the skin at night is beneficial. Massage should always be with outward strokes towards temples.

Another home-made method for removing shadows is as follows:

Wrap oat flour and dust of sandalwood in a napkin. Soak it in unheated milk or rose water and rub on the face.

Pock Marks

A pock-marked face is a curse. Make-up can hide these marks but cannot remove them. There are 2 ways to remove them permanently: (i) Sand-paper surgery and (ii) Skin-peeling. Sand-paper surgery is generally done in foreign countries. It is not prevalent in India due to its exhorbitant cost. The patient has to suffer a lot of pain due to numerous small operations on the skin. These operations are done only by a specialist. For skin-peeling, many kinds of pastes are applied on a patient's face. A layer of skin gets peeled off after application of every paste. The skin gets spotless after repeating the process many times.

Small-pox spots get reduced with age, from childhood to adolescence and growth of the body. Women must look after their skin, specially their face. At night, before sleeping use a deep cleansing-milk and apply nourishing cream. Facials also reduce these spots. Soyabean paste fills the deep spots. Apply soyabean paste on the face. Let it dry for 15-20 minutes, then wash it with lukewarm water. Repeat this thrice a week.

White Spots

White spots or patches on the body is a disease. It is known as leukoderma. This is not a contagious disease. Imbalance of melanin in the body results in appearance of white spots. These patches are directly related to the nature of the skin. Darker skin has more patches because such skin carries more melanins. It must be clarified that white patches are neither congenital nor hereditary. Children are not affected if the mother has these patches. It is erroneous to think that a woman with leukoderma will not be able to lead a normal life. Generally, doctors recommend a solution of carbolic acid to be applied around the spots to prevent them from spreading. Ayurvedic medical science practitioners recommend bawachi oil massage and in many cases the repeated massaging brings the skin to its normal colouring. Natural therapy can also be used as a remedial measure but it is costly. Make-up helps in hiding these spots temporarily. Apply 'foundation' after thoroughly cleaning the skin. It is very important to note that the colour of the 'foundation' should be darker than the colour of your skin. Now apply face powder and make-up as per your wish. At night it is useful to apply calamine lotion after removing the make-up completely.

Sun-Burn or Tanning

Sun-rays are very important for keeping the skin healthy, but sun-burn can be extremely harmful for the skin. As you already know, Sun is a big bowl of fire from which many kinds of rays emanate. We can see the rays of light but we cannot see the infra-red and ultra-violet rays, which are also present. Infra-red rays are hot and bring warmth to the body. Ultra-violet rays provide vitamin 'D' to the body, which is essential for our health. But the skin gets burnt due to excess ultra-violet rays. Melanins, underneath the skin, prevent the skin from getting burnt, that is why the blondes or the dark-complexioned people get less sun-burns than the fair-complexioned people. This is because the darker the skin, more the quantity of melanins in the body. Fair-complexioned people are adversely affected by sun-rays. The ill-effects of sun-rays are the most on children between 6-8 years of age, on women between 25-30 years of age and on men between 30-35 years of age. Ultra-violet rays destroy the melanins in the body and the skin darkened. The rays cut and crack the skin. It results in dryness of the skin. As a result, the skin swells and rashes appear. In such situation fresh melanin comes out and the skin gets blackened.

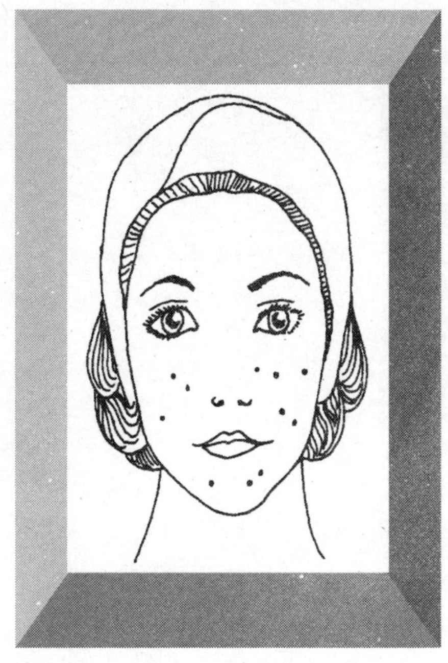

Sun-burn affects the body in the same way as does the burning by steam or hot oil. It results in dryness of skin swelling of blood vessels and damage to cells. Ordinary sun-burn can be cured within 3-4 days but a strong sun-burn causes rashes and the skin peels-off in layers. Obviously, new cells grow and a new skin does appear again but it is drier and thicker as compared to the original one. New skin is often brownish in colour, it cracks and wrinkles easily and such wrinkles are hard to cure. You may benefit from a cold water bath if you are suffering from sun-burn, but avoid using soap. It is specially advisable to take a shower-bath. Coconut oil, cold cream or antiseptic cream should be applied on the dried skin. Lacto-calamine is also beneficial. If it is a mild sun-burn wash it with cold water and apply any antiseptic cream. Remember to protect the skin from sun until the sun-burnt area gets cured. If rashes appear again consult a specialist. The degree of tolerance of sun rays depend upon the nature of the skin. Direct sun-rays are harmful in the month of June when the sun gets nearest to the Earth. Sun-rays are dangerously hot between 12 noon and 2 o'clock in the afternoon. Drink as much lemon-water (nimbu-pani) as you can during this period of the day for a cooling effect.

5. UNWANTED FACIAL HAIR

Unwanted hair, especially on the face, should be a matter of great concern to a woman. There can be many reasons for this unwanted growth like congenital cause, imbalance of hormones, pregnancy, irregular menses, mental tensions, long illness, worries and shocks. One should immediately remove unwanted hair when they begin to grow, instead of just feeling embarrassed. In the medical terminology it is called 'hirsutism'. Unwanted hair grows mostly on the chin, on the upper lip and on the forehead. Most women suffering from hirsutism are in the age group of 15-25. There are many ways to get rid of unwanted hair. For example, plucking, threading, waxing, etc. Since the main reason for unwanted hair is the imbalance of hormones inside the body, it is imperative to get it treated medically. The first step in the medical treatment is a thorough check-up. In case of some defect in the uterus, it is treated by an operation.

Electrolysis is the only permanent treatment for removing facial hair. This treatment has gained wide popularity in India.

Electrolysis

Electrolysis, as a means of permanently removing unwanted hair, was first introduced by Dr Charles Michael in 1857. In 1916, this treatment acquired prominence among the various methods of enhancing beauty. In this process, the roots of the hair are

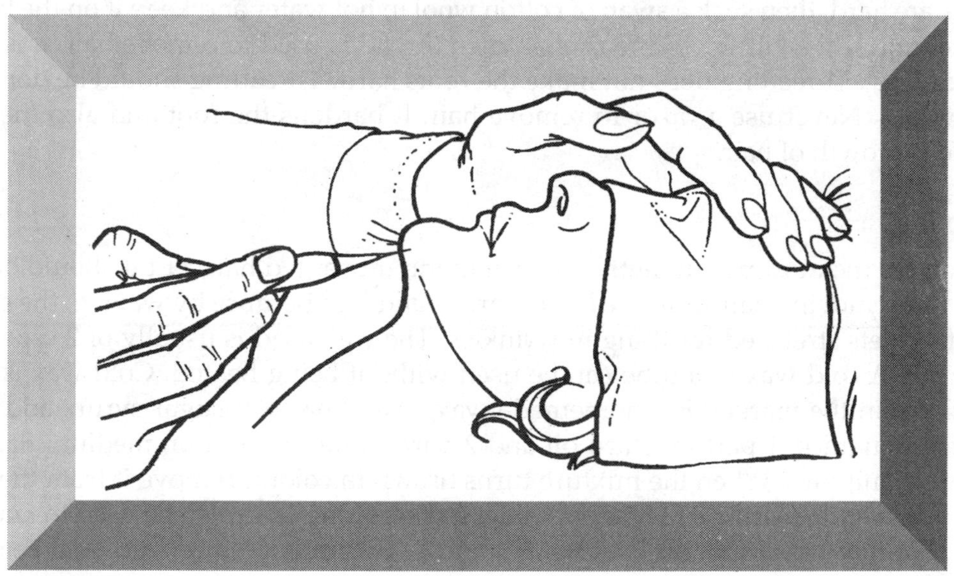

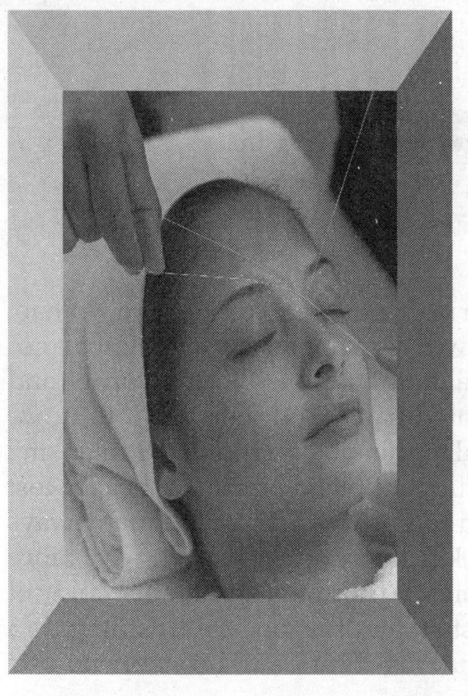

weakened by subjecting them to electric currents. Repeated treatment stops their growth. There are two methods electrolysis. One is 'Galvanic multiple needle method' and the other is 'short-wave method'. In India, the short-wave method is popular. It takes very little time to remove hair by this method and only one needle is used. But it is important to understand that electrolysis should be done only by an experienced beautician. In order to make the area insensitive or dead, 'zylokin' is rubbed as an anaesthesia and then the slanted needle is pricked till the root of the hair. The thickness of hair decides the depth of the needle to be pricked. Then the roots of the hair are burnt by using electric current. Electrolysis should not be used to remove hair from the eyelashes, inner side of the nose and ear and from the pimples. Do not opt for electrolysis if you are being treated by a doctor for hormoned deficiency or for diabetes.

Plucking (Threading)

If there is 1 or 2 unwanted hair on the face, then it should be pulled out by a tweezer. This pulling of hair by a tweezer is known as 'plucking'. If there are a lot of hair then do not use tweezer because the root gets hardened and repeated pulls may result in injury to the root of hair and subsequent growth of pimples and acne. Before using a tweezer apply cold cream to the face so as to soften the roots of the hair. In case the roots are hard, then soak a swab of cotton wool in hot water and keep it on the hair for some time. This will soften the roots. When thread is used to remove hair, it is called 'threading'. Threading does not make the roots hard. Threading should be done after 2-3 weeks. Never use a razor to remove hair. It hardens the root and also there is a rapid regrowth of hair.

Waxing

Waxing is the most useful method of removing unwanted hair, but it should be used only for removing hair from the hands, arms, and legs because by waxing, the skin on the face gets stretched resulting in wrinkles. The wax used is usually of 2 types, cold and hot. A cold wax in a tube can be used without being heated. Cold wax is easily available in the market. For homemade wax, take 8 parts of sugar syrup, add to it 1 part lemon juice, 1 part mustard oil and 2 parts water. Heat it on medium flame for about 45 minutes. When the mixture turns brown in colour, remove it from the flame and add a little glycerine to it and then let it cool. Honey can also be used to make hot wax. For this take 5 spoonfuls of honey. Add 1 spoonful of lemon juice and heat it for

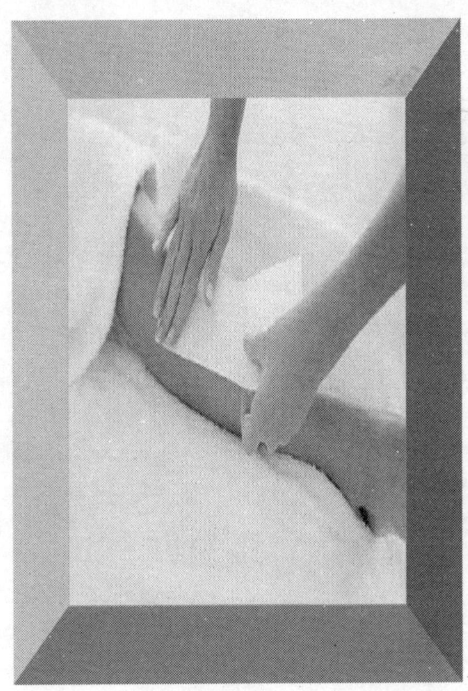

30 minutes on medium flame. Remove it from the heater and add a little glycerine. Let it cool.

The skin must be cleaned by a cleansing-cream before waxing. You may use unheated milk in case cleansing cream is not available. Creamy milk should not be used because it further accentuates the growth of unwanted hair. Use a clean towel to wipe the skin, and while spraying talcum powder, massage it very gently. If the thick roots of hair cause pain, then use cold cream massage before waxing. This will soften the roots. Using a knife, apply hot wax on the skin towards the direction of the growth of hair. Use a thin cloth as bandage on it so that the cloth sticks to the skin. Now pull the cloth with a jerk in opposite direction of the roots of hair. The hair will stick to the cloth and will come out with the root. The container containing the wax should be kept in a utencil full of warm water so that the wax remains hot and in molten condition during the process. Waxing should always be done in an air-conditioned room or under a fan, otherwise the wax will not stick to the hair, due to sweat. Even cooler does not help as the moisture from it prevents the waxing process. Immediately after waxing, the skin should be lightly massaged with lanolin-cream or skin-tonic. This will make the skin smooth and silky.

6. BLEACHING

Strong winter winds and scorching summer heat are natural enemies of complexion. Beauty-conscious women feel concerned over the ravages of weather and seek timely help of beauticians. Bleaching is useful in regaining the original complexion and helps in revitalising the paleness of skin caused due to heat or dryness. It also prevents growth of facial hair. Generally, threading or waxing is advised as a remedial measure for removal of unwanted hair. Waxing leads to wrinkles and threading hardens the roots of the hair. Bleaching, on the other hand, colours the thin and fine hair and keeps the complexion fair by hiding these tiny hair.

Often, I get clients with problems arising from faclty bleaching at home. In an attempt to bleach their face themselves, women often do them incorrectly and some what harm their face. Bleaching requires an efficient knowledge of the ratio and proportion of the powder and other ingredients. Different proportion are required for different persons. Disproportionate mixture can harm the skin and cause allergy to bleaching or may scorch the skin making it smudgy. It is, therefore, advisable to get one's first bleaching done by an expert beautician. Later, on learning the technique, one may do it on their own. But, it is better to use a small quantity of the mixture on the sensitive skin on the lower side of the neck to test its effect. If there is minor irritation, you need not worry. But if the burning is sharp, discontinue the use immediately.

Deep cleansing must be done before bleaching. Clean your face and neck with a wet cotton swab to remove all make-up. Eye make-up should be removed by soaking cotton wool swab in rose water. Now, apply the bleaching cream (or paste) on your face and neck with a brush or cotton wool swab. If there is mild burning sensation, go ahead without worrying about it, but if the sting is hard remove the cream (or paste) immediately. A test of 5 minutes duration is enough. Bleach your neck also along with the face, otherwise there will be a marked difference in the colour of your face and neck. Avoid your eyes and eyelashes. Cover you eyes with cotton balls soaked in rose water to prevent the paste from flowing in. Do not bleach if you have pimples or acne. Allow the pack to remain for 10 minutes, then wash off. Dry the skin and apply cold cream on the face and neck massaging lightly. Use of a good astringent lotion can relieve minor burning sensation. Sometimes small red rashes may appear after the paste is washed off. However, this is not serious. So do not panic. These rashes will disappear of their own after a while.

The bleaching paste can be prepared by taking 1 spoonful of bleaching powder, and half a spoon of hydrogen peroxide. Put 2 or 4 drops of ammonia in it, mix well using cotton swab or a brush. Close the lid immediately.

***

7. COMMON PROBLEMS IN TEENAGERS

Pimples

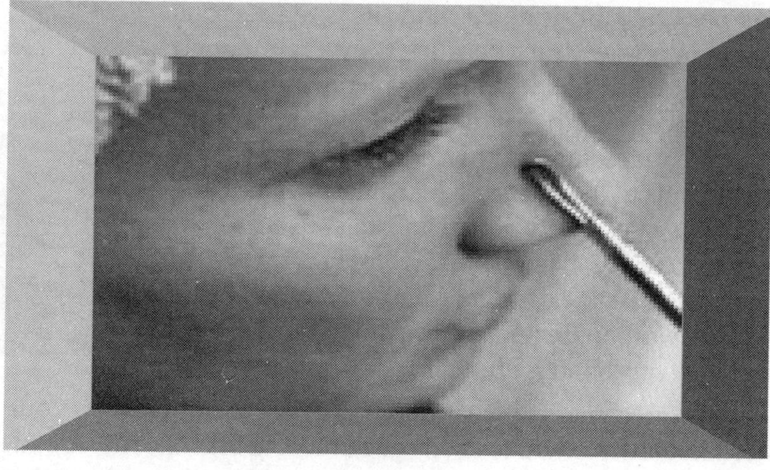

Pimples are a serious adolescence problem. They appear on the cheeks, forehead and nose and spoil your appearance. Why do pimples appear in youth? The answer to this question is simple: As soon as we cross childhood and step into adolescence, different parts of our body begin to develop. The oil-glands underneath the skin become over-active and ooze grease. This grease blocks the pores and pimples sprout. The dust particles clogging in the pores are called 'blackheads.'

A special skin care is essential to guard against pimples. Use of sulphur soap or facewash is effective in keeping the oil glands clean. Grease can be removed by using lemon juice or 'camphor-spirit'. Removing make-up at night, before going to bed, is very important because make-up particles block the pores and prevent them from breathing freely. Steaming once a week keeps the pores open. Multani mud pack is effective in controlling pimples. Peeling-off pimples causes septic and leaves permanent marks. Marks, however, can be subdued to a great extent by applying cucumber juice and rose-water mixture. Pimples can be cured by daily intake of a spoonful of honey mixed with sulphur powder.

Do not neglect pimples. Be alert as soon as they appear. Some people tend to take them lightly because of the old belief that pimples signifies the approach of youth and they will vanish all by themselves with time. I do not agree with these views. Though it is a matter of common knowledge that pimples appear during the transitional years of adolescence and youth due to over-activity of glands, their appearance should not be taken lightly because these may leave permanent marks on the face and damaging your looks.

Blackheads

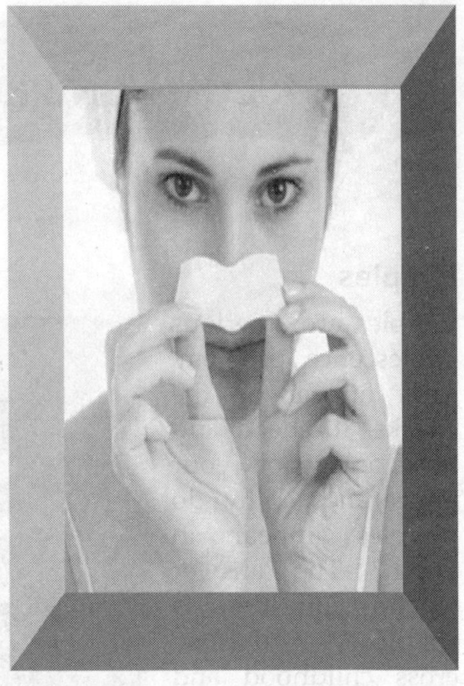

Beauty is a divine gift, and it is our sacred duty to maintain it. But, unfortunately, quacks are doing a great damage to the beauty culture. Taking advantage of the growing beauty consciousness among women, there has been a mushroom growth of the so-called beauty clinics or beauty parlours. Not all of them are run or managed by experts. Most of those who profess to restore your looks are only money-making business, establishments and it is dangerous to fall into their trap, because they are manned by untrained beauticians. I recount here an experience. A couple of days back, a woman with a swollen face came to my clinic. Even her eyes were puffy. On asking, I learnt the disturbing fact that a so-called beautician had used a hair pin to remove blackheads from her face. The experiment caused infection the same evening and the woman developed burning and pricking sensation and had a high temperature.

If you consult a beautician for the treatment of your pimples, make sure, a sterilized instrument is used for removing blackheads. A gadget, known as 'blackhead extractor' is available these days. It should be cleaned regularly and the gadget should be kept in hydrogen peroxide before use.

Acne

Acne is basically a skin disease typical to youth. The skin gets blotchy and these blotches on the face never vanish. Even a beautiful face and smooth skin, if affected by acne, loses its charm. Acne is a deformed type of pimples. Usually, young people pinch the pimples with nails, which results in infection lead to septic. Pimples dry in a couple of days but the marks remain permanent. It is advisable to consult a doctor for acne because it is a kind of skin infection. It may result in pus-pimples due to the presence of infectious bacteria embodied in pimples.

Pus-pimples can be burst with the help of a sterilized needle. The needle is sterilized on a flame and the pimple is pierced to its root. The pus is removed by pressing the sides. A clean cloth should be wrapped around fingers for pressing pimples. Pus should be cleaned with a clean cloth and the affected part should be dabbed with a thin solution of hydrogen peroxide.

Treatment

- Oily skin should be cleaned frequently so that the oily secretion called sebum coming out of the sebaceous glands does not thicken and clog the pores. Acne bacteria breeds fast in greasy spots. Acne can be forestalled through frequent cleanliness.
- Do not scratch pimples with nails even if they are itchy. Scratching may give temporary relief but it may leave permanent mark because nails, howsoever clean, contain bacteria and cause infection. It is advisable to use clean cotton wool swab soaked in hot water to clean pimples.
- Shampoo your hair frequently. Sebaceous glands underneath the hair secrete oil which spreads on the face and give rise to acne. Moreover, long hair touch the face, forehead and neck. If they are clean, the chances of spreading the oil is less.
- Avoid greasy, spicy, fried food. Also minimize the use of sweets, butter, ice-cream and chocolate. Take a balanced diet.
- A sound sleep, morning walk, regular exercise and good bowel movement are other helping agents. Prevent constipation. It gives rise to pimples.
- If affected with acne, avoid heavy make-up. If at all you have to have a make-up, remove it as soon as you can.
- Different types of medicines are available for acne treatment. Anti-biotices, x-rays and ultra-violet rays are effective methods. But, treatment should be undertaken under medical advice.

❋❋❋

8. ENHANCING THE EYES

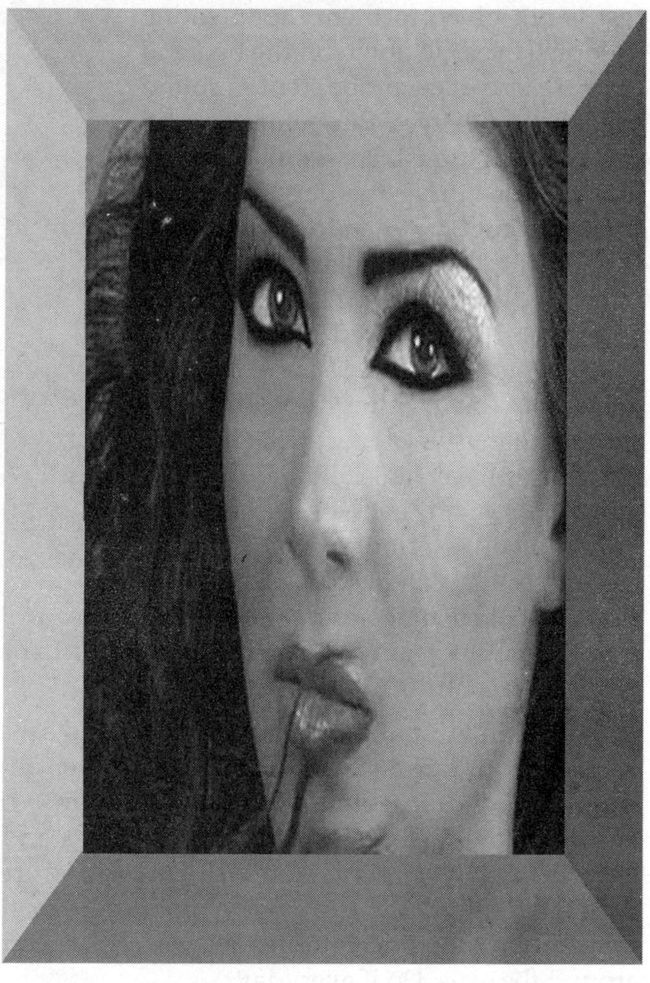

Eyes occupy the most prominent place among the five sensory organs of our body. Large and beautiful eyes enhance one's beauty manifold. There are two kinds of beautiful eyes. One is related to the general health of a person and the second is related to make-up. Healthy eyes are directly related to good health. Loss of vitamins 'A' and 'D' make the eyesight weak. Sometimes weak eyes are hereditary. Never hesitate to use spectacles in case of weak eyesight. Spectacles that complement your face goes a long way in enhancing your beauty rather than diminishing it. If loss of vitamins 'A' and 'D' is the cause of poor eyesight then apart from medical treatment you should take milk, cheese, eggs and green vegetables. For specific problems in the eyes, like conjunctivitis or watery eyes, you should consult an ophthalmologist (eye specialist). Necessary precautions must be taken to keep your eyes healthy. You must see that there is sufficient light while reading, writing or sewing. You must wash your eyes with eyewash once or twice a week. Rose water or water of triphala is very beneficial for the eyes. It brings back the brightness. Even boric powder can be used for washing eyes. Bright light is also harmful. You must use sun-glasses whenever you have to go out in days of strong sunshine. After a hard working day lie down, close your eyes and place on them cotton wool swabs soaked in ice-cold water.

There is one more way to revitalize tired eyes. Placing your elbows on the table, close your eyes with your palms. Allow the weight of your head to fall on the palm. Your eyes require about 8 hours of rest everyday, otherwise they appear heavy. Smoking makes eyes yellowish. Eyes become red if proper rest is not given to them. For treating drooping eyes, lie down on the bed and place a piece of cucumber (cut in round shape) on both eyes. But before this, all eye make-up must be removed. Eyes require rest during the day also, apart from the night. Whenever your eyes feel tired, close them and place your palms on them. You will see darkness and some hazy blurred figures. Open your eyes for some time and again place palms on them. After repeating this process many times, you will find that the figures have vanished and only the darkness remain. Lack of sleep results in dark curcles under the eyes and sometimes the skin becomes flabby. For this, crush a cucumber, wrap it in a thin, transparent cloth and place on the eyes for 10-15 minutes. Doing this twice a week will give great results.

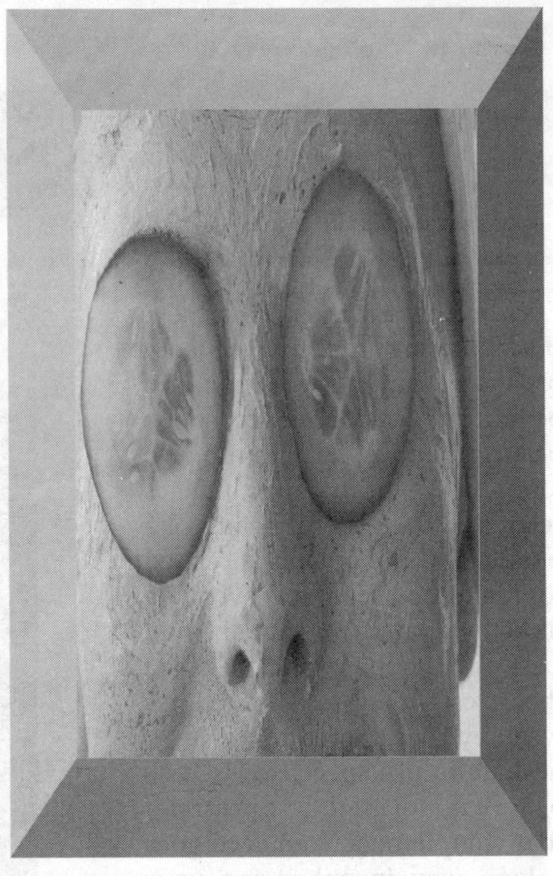

The skin around the eyes is very soft and sensitive. Do not rub your eyes if there is irritation or burning. Do not rub cream, etc., on this surface otherwise the skin will shrink and wrinkles will appear. Apart from wrinkles, many a times dark patches appear below the eyes. When there are folds and creases below the eyes, they have to be treated by surgery. 'Anti-wrinkles cream' are also helpful. To avoid wrinkles or dark spots below the eyes, use almond oil. For this you can also use a home-made preparation. Boil and filter tea-leaves, soak a cotton swab in it and foment the area around the eyes. Do it everyday.

Simple Exercises for the Eyes

- Flickering of eyelashes is an automatic exercise. Close your eyes tightly. Then try to open them as wide as possible. Repeat the process 10 times. During the exercise only flicker the eyelashes, the eyebrows should be kept static.

- Eyeballs should be rotated 20 times to the left and 20 times to the right. Eyelids must remain closed during the rotation.
- Flicker both your eyes simultaneously and speedily. Repeat the flickering after closing the eyes for some time. Repeat this process ten times. Eyeballs get greasy by doing this exercise.
- Look into the mirror for 5 minutes meeting your eyes with the eyes of your reflection in the mirror.
- Mark some far-away object. Look at it for 2 minutes. Then look at some object closer to you. Again look at the far-off object and again look at the nearer object after 2 minutes. Do this exercise for 10 minutes.
- Slowly raise your eyes skywards. Keep them stationary for about 30 seconds. Then again lower them until you can see your feet. Repeat the exercise 15 times.

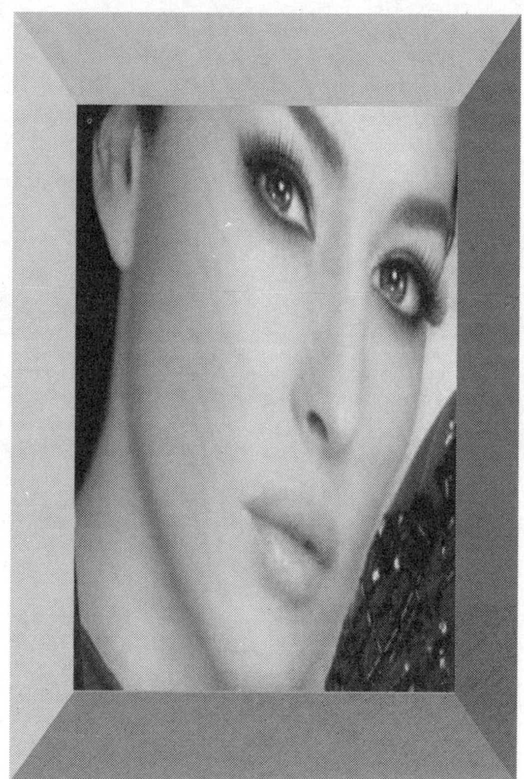

- Take clean, cold water in a broad bowl. Put a little eye-lotion in it. Bend and immerse your eyes in it. Then rotate your eyeballs towards right-left and above and below. Keep flickering the eye-lashes while rotating the eyeballs. Initially, you will find this exercise difficult to perform. However, regular practice will make it easy. By this exercise dust particles get washed off.

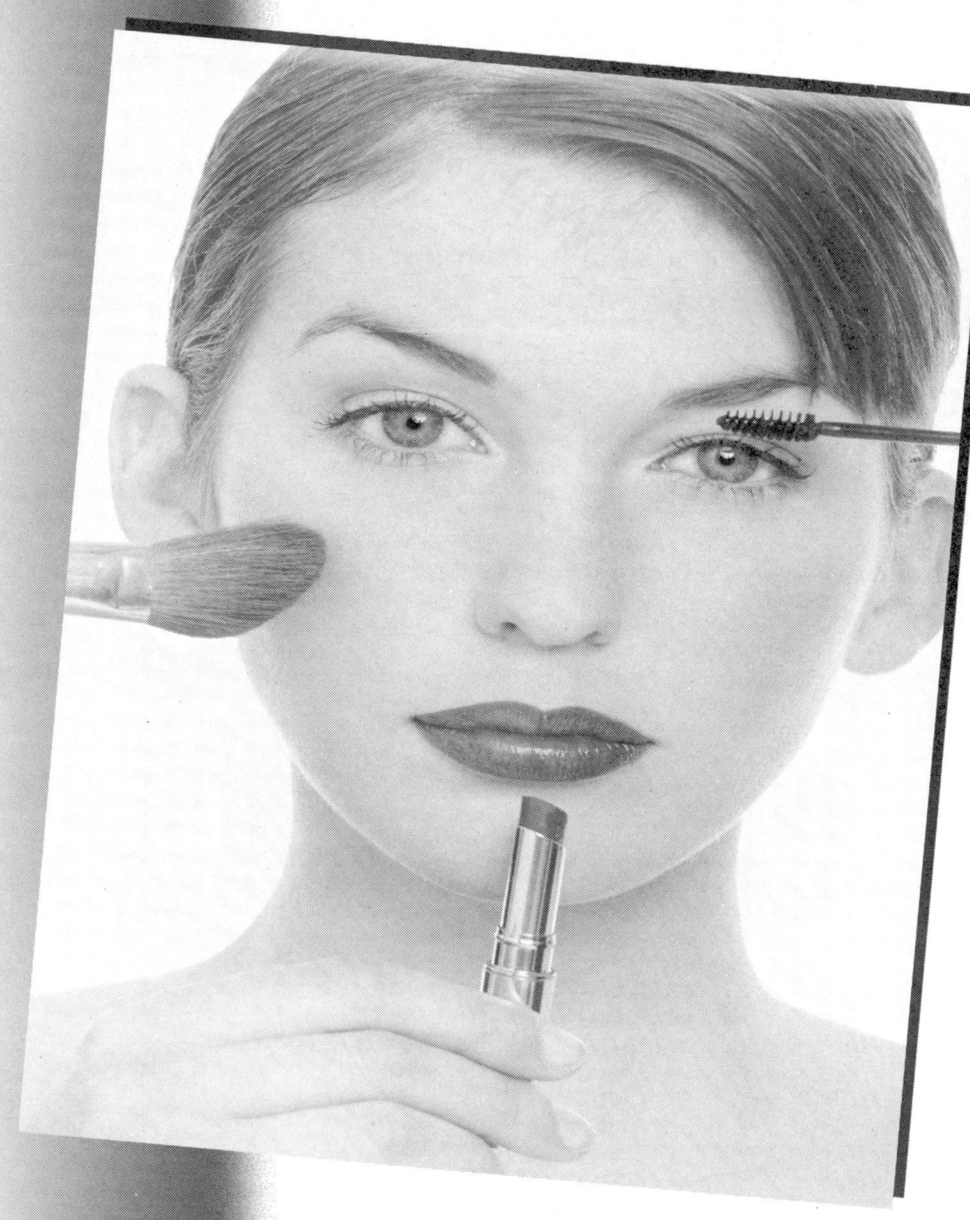

PART 2
MAKE-UP

9. ART OF BEAUTIFICATION

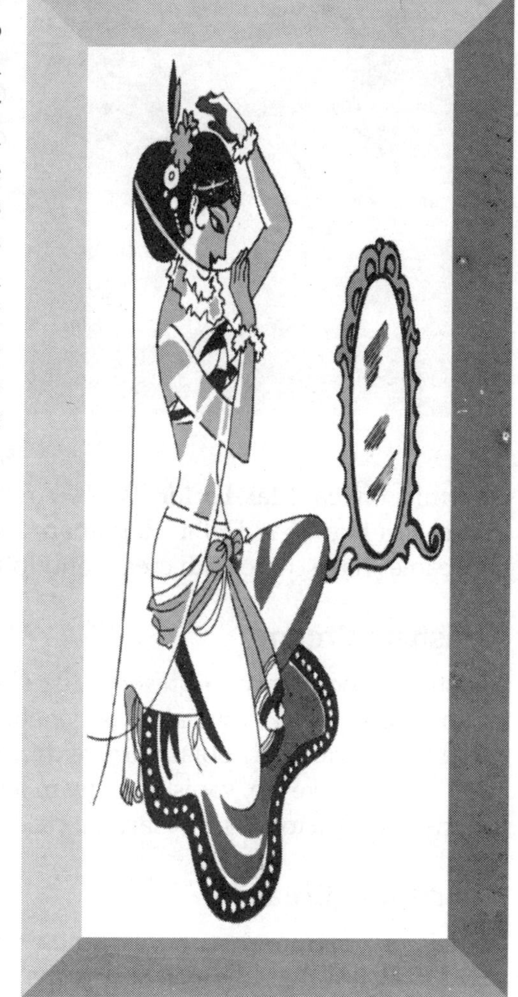

Your face is the most attractive part of your personality. A skillfully done make-up enhances its appeal; it gives you an added dignity in society, and helps you gain self-confidence. But, mind you, make-up should speak for itself, show your taste and enhance your dignity; mere piling-up of beauty aids is not make-up. Unskilled use of cosmetics diminishes natural beauty. There are women who are not beautiful, but because they know how to carry themselves; they able to become the centre of attraction. Attractive personality and beauty are two different things. If you have an appealing personality, your complexion and your looks will add to your charm but, unfortunately, if you have an unattractive personality, only looks will not be able to help you.

A woman should adopt a style of her own so as to stand out in a crowd. It is, therefore, necessary to know the secrets of beauty aids and the art of using them to the maximum advantage. It is also essential to have a thorough knowledge of the various beauty aids available in the market.

It is advisable that for the base, apply a good foundation or lotion on the hands, neck and the face before make-up, so that the skin appears even. Powder gives a kind of glow to the cheeks, so does cream. Rouge heightens the natural pink tinge of the cheeks. Eyes lend charm to the face. Their beauty can be enhanced by make-up.

Although a large number of different beauty aids are manufactured in our country, they should be used according to the specific requirement of one's age, skin, shape of

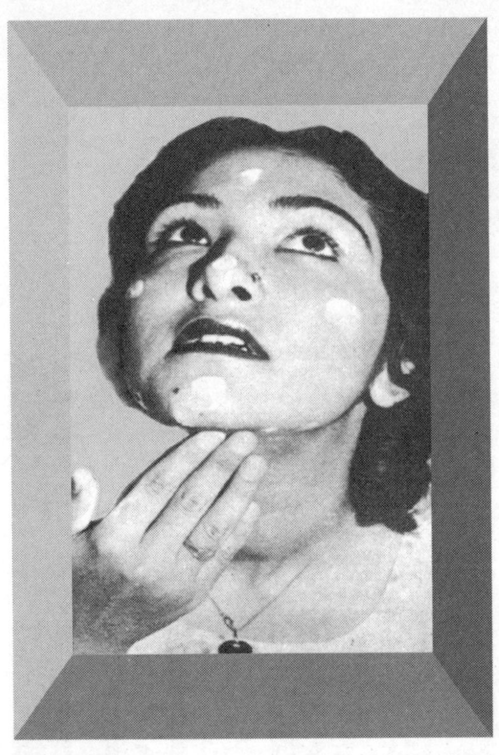

the face, season and occasion. Wrong choice of make-up may adversely impact on your skin; you may look unattractive or more aged than your actual age. In order to keep your facial skin young and glowing you can use various cold creams, vanishing creams, nourishing creams, cleansing creams, astringent lotions, calamine lotions, foundation creams and face powders, but only after knowing which product and brand suits your skin texture.

Cold Cream

Cold cream is used to minimise the effect of the vagaries of the climate. It can also be used as a cleansing cream to clean the skin of dust and dirt. Cleansing creams are made with honey, wax, almond oil, borax powder, rose water and essence. Cold cream can be used all through the year. It protects the skin from the cold biting dry breezes in winter. In the rainy season and in summer, it is used as an all-purpose cream. Some popular brands are: Lakme, Ponds, Charmis, Nivea, Max-Factor, Pears, Afghan Snow, Emami and Johnson & Johnson. In dry places like New Delhi, Rajasthan, UP, it may not suit the weather. In these places companies have come with cream and lotion that suit the weather.

Vanishing Cream

Moisture is necessary to preserve the skin from the ravages of the weather. Vanishing cream keeps the skin moist. It is beneficial for oily and normal skin. Vanishing cream contains stearic acid, potassium hydroxide, glycerine, di-glycol stearate and water. If used before make-up, vanishing cream lends a glow to the face. Some known brands are: Lakme, Max-Factor, Ponds, Garnier, etc.

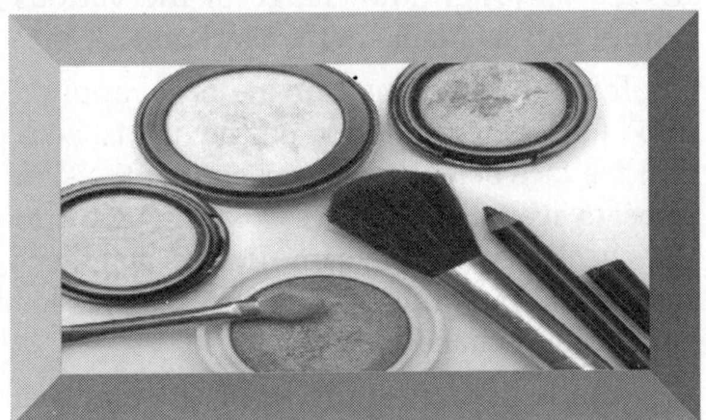

Nourishing Cream

Nourishing cream gives nourishment to the skin. It softens the skin and keeps it glowing. The bottle of nourishing cream should be kept away from the reach of the children because the lanolin, wax and oil contents in it may be injurious to their health. Lakme,

Ponds and Max-Factor are some of the major producers of nourishing creams.

Cleansing Cream

It is used to remove the make-up and dust before going to bed. The layers of make-up, dust and sweat remain as a coat on the face and do not allow the skin to breathe. This results in wrinkles and dullness. Cleansing cream is made of a mixture of stearic acid, mineral oil, lanolin, teropenol, tri-ethanolamine, propyline, glycol and perfume. Some famous brands are : Gala, Lakme, Anne French and Max-Factor.

Astringent Lotion

Astringent lotion is used to check the oily skin's tendency to ooze stickiness, because oil clogs the pores. In order to open them, it is advisable to use a good astringent lotion on the exposed part of the skin. The main ingredients in an astringent lotion are : alum (fitkiri), glycerine and water. Some well-known brands of this lotion are: Max-Factor, Lakme, Gala.

Calamine Lotion

Calamine is used to remove the spots on the skin and to make it even. It is available in various shades according to the requirement of one's complexion. Lakme's Lacto-Calamine and Vicco Turmeric Cream are popular products.

Foundation

Foundation not only disguises the spots, but it also makes the skin smooth so that make-up looks appealing and well-set on the face. Max-Factor's 'Hi-Fi' foundation cream is available in many shades. It can be chosen according to your complexion. 'Satin Glow' by Lakme is in liquid form and is useful for all types of skin. 'Look Natural' by Gala and 'Sheer Genius' by Max-Factor are complete beauty aids in themselves.

Face Powder

Face powder is applied after the application of foundation to make the face look glowing and bright. Face powders are available in different shades and should be chosen according to your skin face. Chemicals such as kaolin, talc magnesium stearate, magnesium carbonate, zinc oxide, yellow oxide, grey oxide and perfume are major constituents of face powders. Care should be taken not to inhale face powder because the chemicals in it are injurious to lungs. These may cause cancer. Lakme, Max-Factor and Ponds are leading manufacturers of face powders.

10. BASIS OF MAKE-UP: FOUNDATION

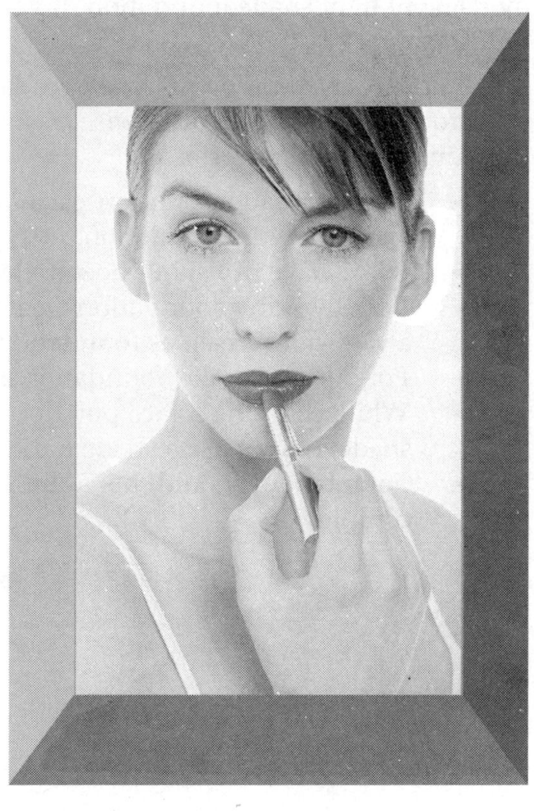

The market is flooded with a large variety of cosmetics which are easily available. It does not require any skill to buy a product, but it does require a thorough knowledge of their different properties. In fact, very few women really know the art of using beauty aids dexterously so as to gain maximum effect with minimum efforts. Foundation creams or lotions play an important role in giving smoothness to the face. Foundation is applied on the facial skin as a base of make-up so as to heighten the glow on the cheeks. Here are some tips on the correct use of foundation in order to make your face look attractive.

Foundation is applied before make-up. First, clean your face with deep cleansing milk. Foundation is not only the base of your make-up, it is also the protecting agent of your skin, as well as an effective medium to hide your pimples, shadows and other spots. The face looks clean, soft and fresh.

Foundation is usually available in the form of a thick cream in a bottle or tube. Take a small quantity on your left palm and apply a little on your face with the fingers of your right hand. Instead of fingers, you can also apply it with a cotton wool swab after dipping it in rose-water. Use it profusely on your neck also, otherwise your neck will look darker than your face. Foundation is applied with an upward motion from the chin onwards with the tips of finger. Thus, it gets absorbed in the skin. Let it dry for a while before starting your make-up. For dry skin, it is necessary to apply glycerine with a cotton wool swab before using foundation. If your skin is oily, use astringent lotion mixed with a drop or 2 of rose-water or lemon juice. Now, apply foundation and make it even by rubbing the face lightly with tissue paper. Also, clean your eye brows and eye lashes of all the extra foundation sticking over them. This cleaning should also be done with a tissue paper.

The shape of your face can be changed to some extent by foundation. If you have a round face, use a dark shade of foundation; for square and diamond shaped face, use a darker shade over the jaw and the chin. If the skin below your eyes has a subdued colour, you can heighten it by using darker shade on the spot. Similarly, shadows and black spots below the eyes can be hidden under a coating of light shade foundation. A broad nose can be made to look thinner if a darker shade is applied on each side of the nose. If you have double-chin then by applying dark shade of foundation on its underneath part it can be made to look balanced. You can make your chin prominent by using of light shade foundation. If your cheek bones are raised, apply dark shade foundation below them.

Take care that you do not use foundation in large quantity. Wash-off your make-up before retiring to bed, otherwise the particles will clog your skin-pores preventing the skin from inhaling fresh air.

- Use foundation only on clean skin. Do not try to give a 'touch' to a stale make-up with foundation.
- If you have dry skin, choose a lanolin mixed foundation cream.
- For oily skin a foundation cream without lanolin is useful. You can also use a vanishing cream as foundation.
- For oily skin 'cake' foundation is good.
- While choosing a face powder, take care to use the same shade or a lighter shade. Do not use a shade darker than the shade of your foundation.
- Foundation should be a little darker than the shade of your natural complexion.

11. APPLYING CREAM THE RIGHT WAY

It is often observed that women apply cream on their faces in large quantities without realising that they are simply wasting it, because piling cream on the face is not enough. Cream is an effective ingredient to keep the skin beautiful and healthy. It covers the skin with its oily crust preventing the cells from developing dryness. Cream should be in commensuration with your skin. So, one has to keep in mind the quality of one's skin—normal, oily or dry. According to the requirement, buy a good product, because sub-standard products, though less expensive, are harmful for the skin. The chemicals used in them or the defective process which goes in their making makes the products unhealthy for usage.

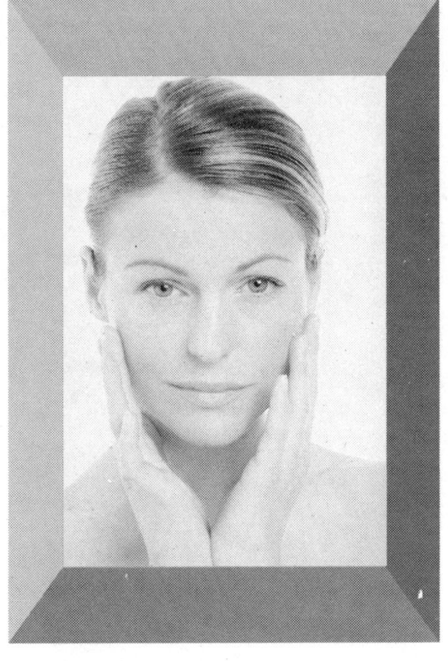

The correct way to apply cream on your face in as follows:

Take cream on your finger, apply it and massage it slowly upwards to the middle portion of your face. Apply it on the forehead and massage from the inward corners of the eyebrows to outwards. Then, from the mid-point of the eyebrows, massaging in circular motion, move down below the eyes. Massage the nose from its upper part to downwards and then to nostrils, from nostrils to the temples. Now, apply cream on the upper lip and move towards the cheeks. Apply below the lower lip and move down till you reach below the chin. In the end, apply below the chin and massage downwards.

Every day after bath, clean your face with a cleansing cream or lotion. It removes dirt and opens the pores. Likewise, it cleans the particles of a previous make-up, and removes other spots, if any. Now when the skin is clean, apply cream and rub it well so that it gets absorbed. Use a non-oily foundation, as far as possible. Cream should be used on the face, neck and on those parts which are exposed. In order to protect the skin from the heat-wave and the scorching summer Sun, use some good sun-screen cream or lotion.

***

12. APPLYING POWDER

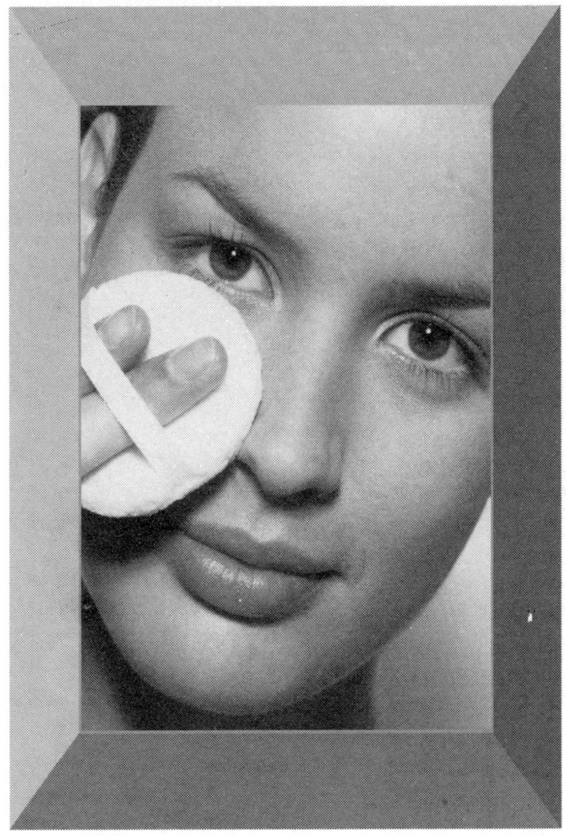

Powder is an effective beauty aid to make the skin look even softer and attractive. Powder is the last item of your make-up. It is available in 2 forms—cake and powder. While choosing a powder, keep in mind your complexion, and choose a shade that goes with it, otherwise the 2 shades, one of your complexion and the other of the powder will not blend. The skin will look blotchy. Do not use cake powder, if you have an oily skin, because it contains an oil-base. While using powder, be sure your locks of hair are not dangling on your face. Apply powder with a clean, cotton puff and discard the used one.

Powder should be dabbed on the face slowly dexterously with a trained and steady hand. When applied with light pressure, it settles down in the pores. Do not forget to use it on the neck. Dust off the extra powder. A powder brush or a cotton wool pad are the best to dust it off. If powder is not well-set, the face looks blotchy. Powder sticks on the eyebrows and eye lashes. Brush it off with an eye brow brush in an anti-clock wise movement (from the end of the eyebrow upwards).

***

13. APPLYING ROUGE

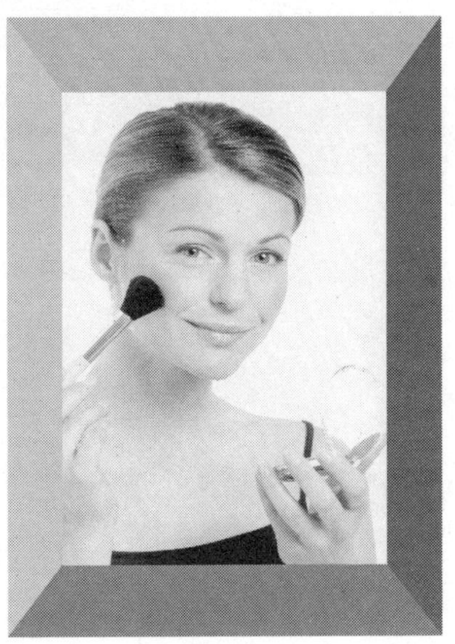

Rouge is applied after applying foundation. Unfortunately, rouge is the most ill-used cosmetic. Many women lack the art of applying rouge effectively; they either apply in excess or too less. An excessive coating dampens natural beauty. Choice of wrong shades or ability to use it effectively spoils the womans look.

Rouge brings glow to an otherwise lustreless cheeks makes them attractive and natural. Rouge should be used as to heighten the natural lustre.

Rouge is available in 3 types — liquid, cream and cake. Liquid and cream rouge is used after applying foundation and before the use of powder, whereas cake rouge is used after the application of powder. Rouge should be of the same tinge as your skin. Fair skin needs lighter tinge whereas dark skin requires deep colours.

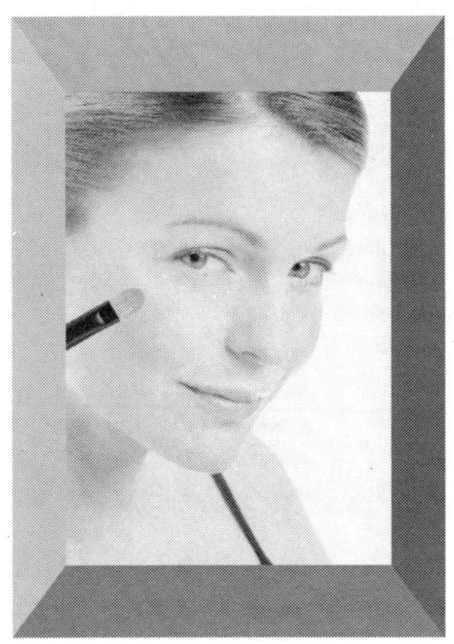

The purpose of applying rouge is to heighten the flush (red or pink glow) on the skin. It is, therefore, necessary that it is applied only on those parts of the face which can naturally flushed. For example, on the cheek-bones, just below the eyes, and towards the end of eyes. Spread it with our fingers after applying it with a brush. Do not put it near the nose which, otherwise would appear short and broad, nor near the eyes. If it is spread below the cheeks, it gives an oldish look. Yes, you can put it on your chin. It, then, gives an oval shape to the face.

***

14. APPLYING LIPSTICK

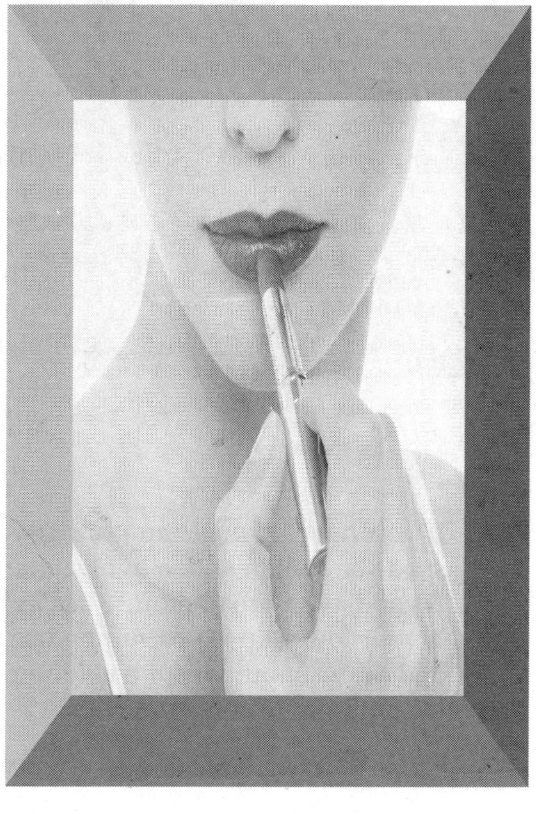

Lipsticks add colour to your lips. Every beauty-conscious woman should be aware of the right shade of lipstick to be used which will complement the shape of her face, lips, complexion and her clothes. Lipstick is considered to be a morale booster, and essentially helps a woman gain self-confidence.

Lipstick is used to add life to the lips but if applied shabbily, it looks ugly. Before applying lipstick clean the lips with a piece of cotton wool swab dipped in cleansing milk. Lipstick does not give lustre if lips are not clean. Do not use soap on the lips because they have soft skin. Apply foundation as a base on the lips then let it dry and apply lipstick by first drawing an outline followed by filling it in. Lipstick can be applied with a brush but it requires skill and practice. If lipstick spreads on apply powder on them, let it dry and then apply lipstick. Many times it is not very comfortable to apply it while standing, because hands may shake and thus it may spread. So, it is advisable to use a dressing-table, rest your elbows on the dressing table. Put on lipstick on the upper lip, followed by the lower lip. Use a lighter tinge first and then darker for glow. After applying a light tinge, keep a tissue paper between your lips and wipe off the extra lipstick with tissue paper. Then use a dark colour. Blend both the colours with a brush. Using a lip gloss adds to lustre to lips after applying lipstick.

Lipstick can change the look of the lips – broad lips can be made to look thin and vice versa and the shape of lips can also be moulded to some extent. If you have a small face use light shade on lower lip and darker tinge on the upper lip. Likewise, apply light shade on the upper lip and dark on the lower lip if lips are thin. For broad lips reduce the out-line considerably. On the contrary for making thin lips look broad enhanse the outline. Uneven lips can be given the desired shape by making

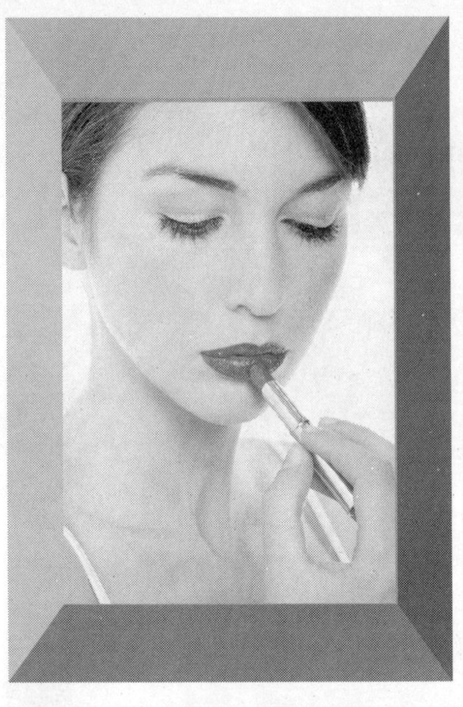

an appropriate outline. For thickness apply two coats. Remove the lipstick before going to bed. It is advisable to use a good quality product; sub-standard product can spoil the colour and texture of your lips.

Choose the lipsstick shade as per your age, the occasion and the clothes you are wearing. Natural shades suit young girls. Working women should not use bright shades while going to work. Young women with fair complexion between 18-25 should use pink shades. Women with dark complexion in this age group can use broken shades. Women between 25-40 should go in for lighter shades.

As for the colour of outfit you wearing, like with orange shade of your sari, use pink lipstick, with pink sari use crimson. You cannot match you lipstick with every outfit that you wear, but you can always wear something that complements your skin tone.

Tips

- If you have a small mouth, draw outer outline with a lip pencil of a darker shade and fill in with a light shade lipstick.
- If you have a broad mouth, use light shaded lipsticks.
- If your lower lip is protruding use dark shade lipstick at the centre of your lips and draw an outline with a lighter shad.
- Do not re-touch on a stale lipstick. It does not shine. Nor does it look even.

15. BEAUTIFYING YOUR EYES

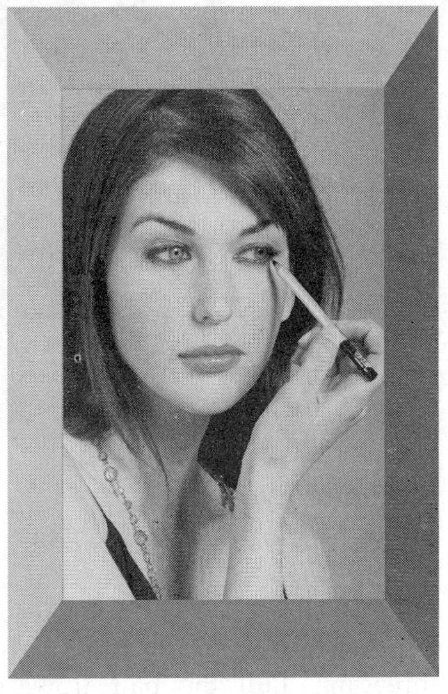

You are lucky if you have beautiful eyes — large, twinkling and shapely. But, if you have not been bestowed with this blessing, do not be disheartened. You can enhanse the beauty of your eyes by a few careful strokes here and there. The materials you require are — an eyebrow pencil, eye-liner, eye-shadow and mascara. An eyebrow pencil is used to give shape to eyebrows. But since most Indian women have dark and thick eyebrows they do not generally require a shape. Those with thin or scattered eyebrows can use an eyebrow pencil to make them look shapely.

Eye Make-up

An eye-liner is a liquid used on the eyelashes in a thin line. For small eyes draw a thick line. In eye make-up, the sequence followed is "eyeshadow", eye-liner and mascara.

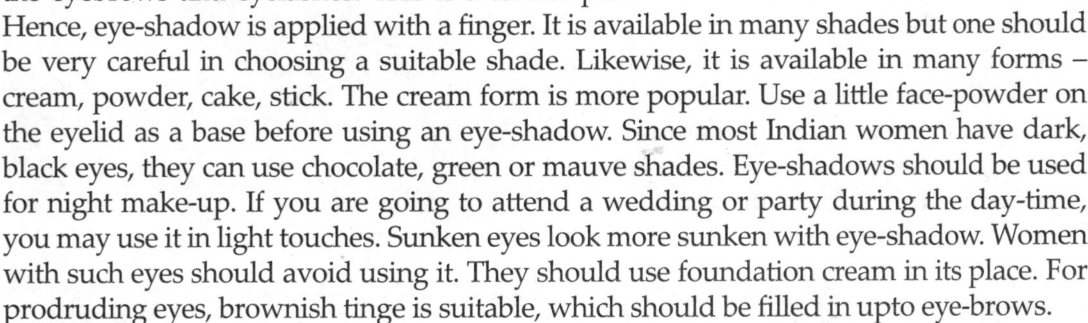

Eye-shadow is used on the eyelid between the eyebrows and eyelashes. This is a tender part. Hence, eye-shadow is applied with a finger. It is available in many shades but one should be very careful in choosing a suitable shade. Likewise, it is available in many forms – cream, powder, cake, stick. The cream form is more popular. Use a little face-powder on the eyelid as a base before using an eye-shadow. Since most Indian women have dark, black eyes, they can use chocolate, green or mauve shades. Eye-shadows should be used for night make-up. If you are going to attend a wedding or party during the day-time, you may use it in light touches. Sunken eyes look more sunken with eye-shadow. Women with such eyes should avoid using it. They should use foundation cream in its place. For prodruding eyes, brownish tinge is suitable, which should be filled in upto eye-brows.

Mascara is used to thicken the eyelashes. It should also be used for evening make-up. Mascara is put on with a brush at the root of the eyelashes and is applied upto the end of the lashes. It is available in many shades, though black is more popular. During day-time, apply black or steel-grey shades. At night, black eye-liner, dark mascara and white eye-shadow is normally used. For bluish and brown eyes, black-eye-liner

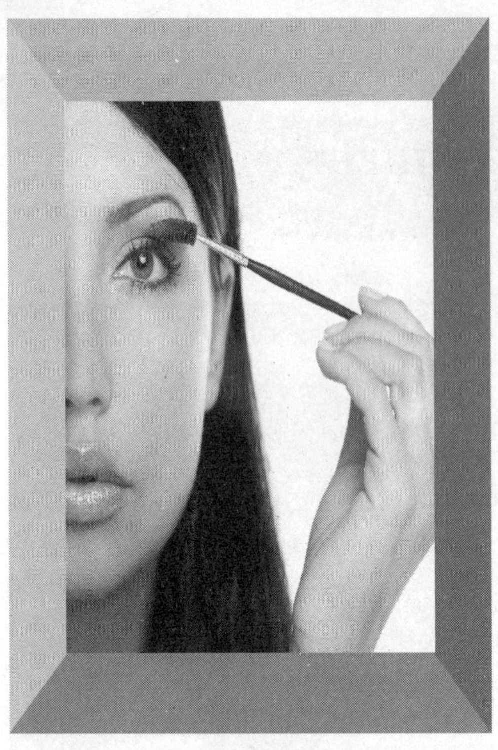

with light blue mascara for day time; and for evenings, blue eye-liner, blue mascara and blue eye-shadow is suitable.

Take care to remove this make-up before going to bed. It should be cleaned with baby oil. Close your eyes, apply baby oil on a cotton wool swab and scrub slowly, gently. First clean the upper part and ends. Open your eyes and clean the lower part.

Some women are allergic to eye make-up. In this case, the eyes redden, water and the skin around the eyes get a burning sensation. Use only good quality products. The markets are flooded with sub-standard or imitation products. Beware of them or you will spoil even your natural charm in a bid to heighten it artificially. Discontinue the use if you feel any irritation, rashes, etc. Always take care to clean your hands and brushes well to avoid infection.

Shape of Eyebrows

Eyebrows play an important role in heightening the beauty of the eyes. Do not give shape to your eyebrows by using a razor, instead, use a plucker or go for threading. Pull the hair upwards from their roots if you are using a plucker pincer. Threading, however, is more advisable to plucking because when plucked with pincers the roots become harder and hard hair sprout. Not so in threading. After plucking or threading use 'Eav-de-cologue' or an anti-septic cream/lotion to prevent a burning sensation.

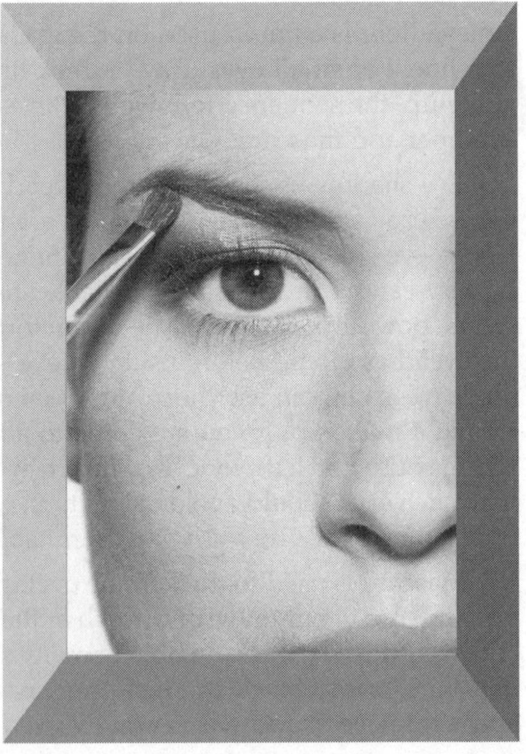

Plucking or threading should start with a point near nose and end towards the outer end of the eyes. First pluck the hair on the sides, then come to the middle lower part. It ensures a good curve. Eyebrows should not be too bushy. They should be thick in the middle and thin and bent at the ends. A drop or two of oil, rubbed gently gives them lustre.

Give shape to your eyebrows according to the shape of your face to enhance the beauty of the face.

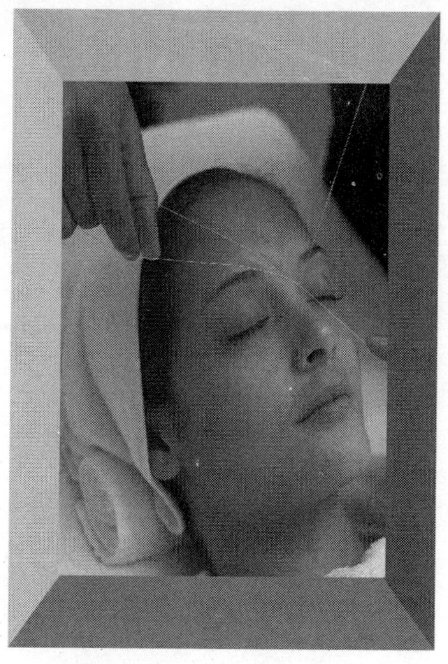

Eyebrows that Suit the Shape of your Face

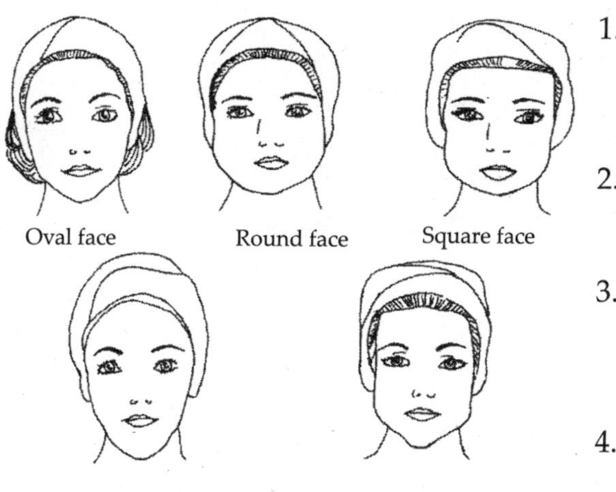

1. An oval face requires small eyebrows (approx. as long as the length of eyes), with trim ends and thick middle.
2. Round face should have long eyebrows with thin ends sliding downwards.
3. On a square face they should be small, crescent-shaped and sliding from both sides. They should be thick and bent at the middle.
4. For a triangular face, have eyebrows which are thick and straight. One-third of the end should bend down.
5. A pearshaped face looks beautiful with straight eyebrows, not very long, but having pointed ends.
6. If you have a longish nose, do not draw eyebrows too high up the eyes otherwise eyes will look very small.

16. BINDI: THE SHINNING STAR

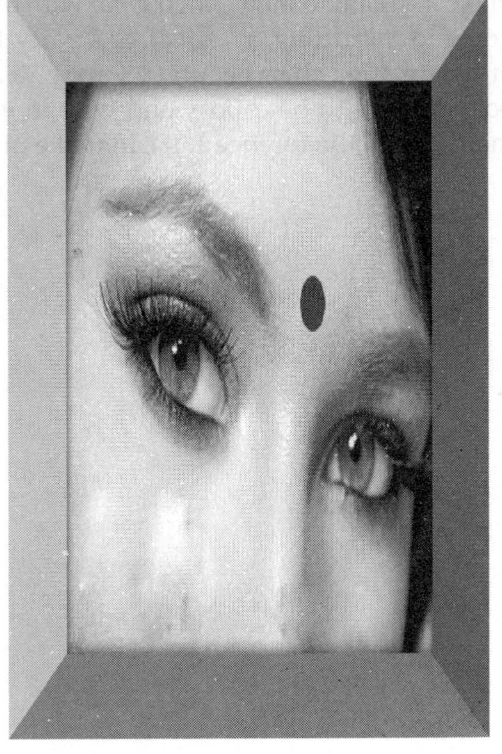

Add a zero to the figure 1 and its value will increase 10 times. Likewise, place a *bindi* (dot) on your forehead after make-up and the charm of the face will enhance 10 times. *Bindi* (also called bindiya) is a symbol, not only of beauty is an indication of a married woman. A married Hindu woman uses various symbols — sindur, bangles, mangal sutra, bichhuye on the toes and 'alta' on the feet. Likewise, *bindi* is a symbol of good luck and purity. It has found its way in folk-literature, poetry, sculpture and other forms of arts and literature.

In ancient times *bhasm* (sacred ashes) or *chandan* (sandalwood paste) were used on the forehead by men. Women decorated the forehead with a red dot symbolic of good luck like the rising Sun. They used materials varying from roli, kumkum, sindur. Today, bindis are available in different colours to match your make-up and dress. Although, traditionally only a round dot is permissible, these days the *bindis* are available in many shapes, some of them being religious symbols like trident (trishul), conch (shankh), star (tara), lamp (deepak) and so on. Today even unmarried women wear *bindi*.

The colour of your dress and the shape of your face should determine the shape, size and colour of the *bindi* you choose. Some popular motifs available are — round, long, oblong, triangular, crescent moon, a round *bindi* with small dots surrounding it, etc. You are the best judge to decide what suits you. Some tips are, however, given here. A small forehead appears large with an oblong *bindi*. A broad forehead looks good with a round *bindi*. On a fair complexion, red looks striking whereas on dark complexion pink, orange or sandalwood colour appears prominent. Whitish complexion requires a light red *bindi*. If the skin is very dark, do not use red, steel grey or chocolate colours. For large eyes, big *bindi* is suitable, for small eyes a small *bindi*.

Height and shape of the body are also determining factors. For example, a tall woman should use round shaped *bindi*, a short woman should put on longish-shaped *bindi*. If you have a broad forehead, place the *bindi* in the middle, but if you have a narrow forehead put it between the eyebrows. In summers, light-tinged *bindi* looks pleasant; in winters and at night bright colours appear prominent. For middle-aged women it is advisable to use deep colours which lend gravity and soberness to their personality.

Bindi can be in liquid or cream form. Powder *bindi* is difficult to use and requires cream or vaseline as base. Glass, lac or plastic *bindis* can be stuck with a little spit. Some women make it a point to match their *bindi* with their attire, irrespective of the fact whether they are going to a wedding, a festival, or a party. But, this is an erroneous attitude, because instead of heightening their beauty, a wrong decision can make you ridiculous and uncultured. So, you have to be choosy and wise in your choice of *bindi*. A *bindi* is much more than a mere dot on the forehead. It can make or mar your charm.

17. PRE-BRIDAL MAKE-UP

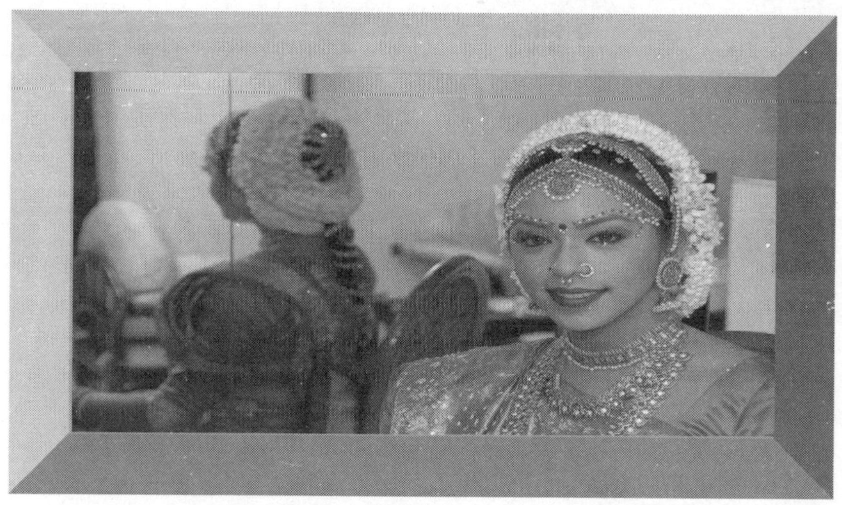

Every woman wants to look beautiful on her wedding day. She would, however, be disappointed if she were to depend on cosmetics to bring sudden changes in her. Cosmetics may, at best, hide a few defects but they do not have the capacity to change your looks. It is, therefore, important that you look after yourself at least 2 months prior to the D-day. Facial once a week will clear the complexion within 2 months. If your town has no facility of a beautician, make face-packs at home and use them. But, do not forget to put cotton wool swabs soaked in rose water on your eyes.

Massage your face lightly with deep-cleansing milk before going to bed. Regular massage gives a natural glow to the skin, because massaging helps in proper blood circulation which, in its turn, makes the skin soft, healthy and attractive. After deep-cleansing, apply nourishing cream and massage lightly. In the morning, sprinkle icy-cold water. Avoid use a soap if the skin is dry. It will crack and leave white patches. Instead, use moisturizer. If the skin is oily, make a paste with oat flour, add lemon juice and rub well. It will prevent pimples.

One month before the wedding stop using make-up. But, if you cannot avoid it sometimes, then clean it off soon. Moreover, stop eating fried food. Drink honey-mixed lemon water first of all in the morning before taking any other drink.

Beautiful hands symbolise a good character. For the beauty of hands remember three things—skin should be soft, fingers should have a beautiful shape, and nails should be well-trimmed. So, stop household works, like cleaning utensils, washing clothes, brooming. Or if you must, then use rubber gloves. Massage fingers with cold cream or cuticle cream at night. After kitchen work, dip fingers in soap water. A home remedy for soft hands is given below:

Take a spoonful of sugar and juice of a lemon on your palm and rub them together with your palms till sugar melts. Honey can replace sugar, if available. It is more effective. This should be done daily for a month before wedding.

It is essential that you are ready with all the required items of make-up two days before wedding so that you remain free of tension. Go to bed early to avoid mental tension. In fact, mental peace enhances natural beauty. If you find it difficult to have a sound sleep, drink a glass of hot milk.

18. BRIDAL MAKE-UP

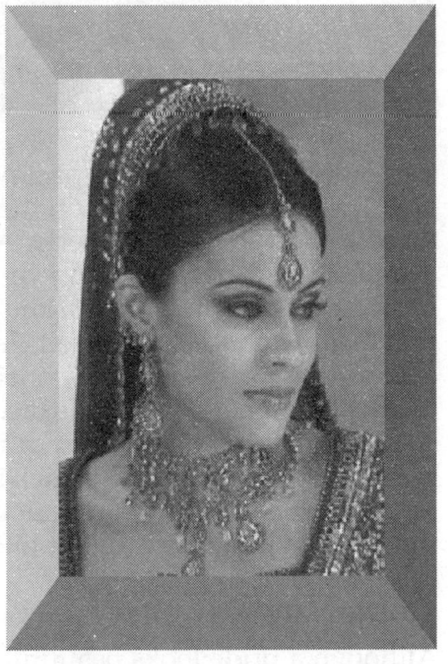

Bridal make-up depends much on the bride's sisters, sisters-in law and her friends because a bride does not decorate herself on her D-day. Nowadays, most brides visit a beauty parlour to get ready. Every woman, therefore, must have knowledge of bridal make-up and of things required for it, because beauty clinics are not available in small towns or villages.

For an immaculate make-up, a soft, smooth and lustrous skin is essential, and hence a couple of weeks before the wedding great care should be taken. Home-made concoction called ubtan, and a good facial give the required softness to the skin. Blackheads can be easily removed by steaming. For a fresh look, use some skin tonic or astringent lotion.

In the morning on the wedding day make nails soft by dipping them in lukewarm water mixed with soap and soda bicarb. Rub nails with a filler to give them the desired shape. The dead skin on the nails can be pushed back with a nail-pusher or an orange stick, after applying olive oil on that part. Cut-off the dead skin with scissors. Massage the arms with cream. Wash hands with lukewarm water and apply hand lotion so that they get a soft and smooth look. Polish nails with nail-polish. Decorate your hands with mehandi just one day prior to the wedding day.

Now, scrub feet and apply 'alta' or *mahawar.* One can visit a parlour for 'manicure' and 'pedicure' one day prior to the wedding, if possible.

Hairstyling

A good hairstyle can be done only if the hair is not oily. So, shampoo them before that. Put them in rollers when wet and then dry them. Long hair as well as short hair both can be put in rollers. Remove rollers when hairs are dry. They will be wavy, and can be set well. Now, draw forth smaller locks and do 'back combing'. Part your hair from the middle and make waves on both sides. A bride can go parting at the for centre which will help her match the tikka. After setting the front hair, tie a beautiful bun. For short hair, you can use ready-made 'switch'. Hair spray will set the hair well and lend them lustre.

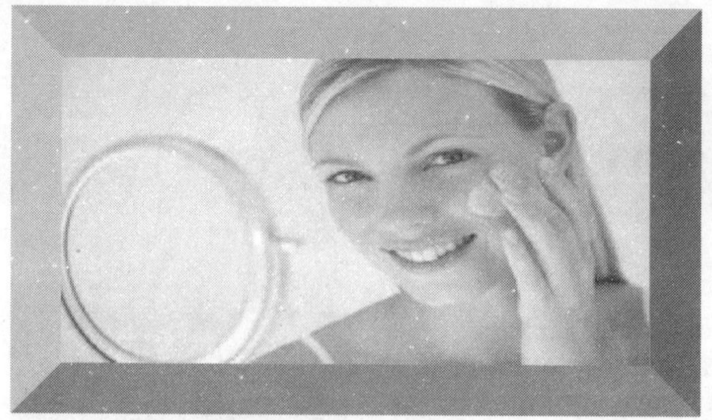

Facial Make-up

Clean the face and use a base cream and then foundation. If there are spots or shadows, hide them by applying light-tinged foundation or concealer on that part. Do not forget to apply foundation on the neck otherwise the neck will appear darker than face. Now put liquid rouge with a brush on the upper part of the cheeks and rub it down gently, it gives a flush to the bride's face. Apply compact powder or face powder evenly so that it does not show in patches. Apply powder on the upper part of eyelids and on lips. Powder holds the mascara and lipstick properly. After face, go for eye make-up: Mascara for eyelids, eye-liner on the lashes and eye-shadow matching the clothes of brides. Maroon or brown eye shadow will suit the bride if she is weaing red dress. Green and golden eye-shadow can also be used depending on the colour of her outfit. Give shape to eyebrows with an eyebrow pencil. Put a *bindi* on the forehead – it could be round or according to the shape of the face. *Bindi* can be red, or any colour that is matching the colour of the dress. Forehead can be decorated with small dots above the eyebrows in the shape of half moon. Lipstick is put on last of all. Apply a light shade first followed by a darker shade. On the lipstick, apply a lip-gloss, to ensure lustre. After completing this process use an astringent lotion so that the make-up stays for long.

Clothes and Jewellery

Although a bride looks beautiful in a red outfit, the colours do vary as per provincial traditions. Moreover, they can be different in style; sari, salwar-kamiz, lehanga-chunni, etc. Golden decorations on a red outfit gives it a kind of glitter. Make-up is not complete without jewellery. *Beni* on the forehead, *zhoomer* or *matha-patti, nath* on nose, earrings, necklace, bangles, *kangans, baju-band*, rings, *hathfool, payal* and so on can be worn.

Aids for Bridal Make-up

- Cleansing milk, cream, astringent
- Foundation, powder, liquid rouge, mascara, red and white bindi, eyeshadow, eye-liner, eyebrow pencil
- Nail polish, lipstick, lip-gloss
- Nail filer, nail push, orange stick, hand lotion
- Mehandi (henna), 'alta' or mahavar
- Blackheads extracter, hairpin, rollers, switch, hair spray, etc.
- Wedding costume, ornaments and jewellery

***

19. BEAUTY IS SKIN DEEP

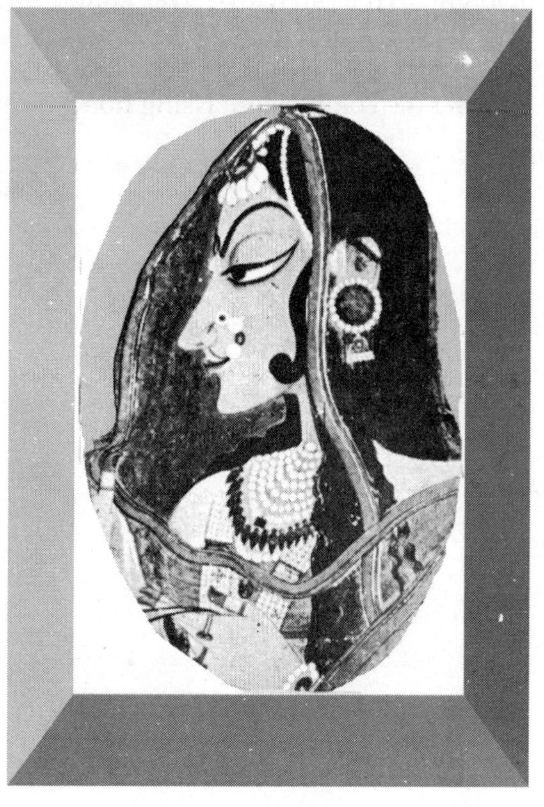

In our country, the measuring rod for a woman's beauty is her complexion. Though theoretically everybody agrees that not complexion, but charm is the most desirable quality of beauty, the deciding factor still is fairness of skin. A healthy, smooth and glowing skin makes a woman stunningly attractive despite her darkish complexion. A fair complexion is prone to pimples, blackheads, spots and shadow. A tasteful make-up and choice of clothes enhance the beauty of a dark woman.

Use liquid foundation before make-up. Select a darker shade of foundation in order to subdue the unwanted glow because a dark skin has a tendency to shine. Moreover, a lighter shade is unsuitable because the face may look patchy. If you are unable to get the correct shade, add a little distilled water in it. Rub in the lotion well so as to absorb it in the skin otherwise after some time, the foundation will appear in waves on the face. Use only a little powder because a darkish complexion requires very less quantity of powder. Almond-brown mascara and light-tinged eye-shadow are more suitable. In the choice of lipstick, go in for a shade lighter than the colour of your lips and give it a light touch. Do not apply profusely. Use any lip-gloss during day time; for evening make-up, use an almond-red shade on your lipstick, but avoid coffee colour shade or pink shade. For dark lips, lip-gloss is good.

Selection of Clothes and Jewellery

A dark woman should avoid black, blue, pink, light brown and sky blue colours. Instead, orange, red, white and yellow colours will suit them. If you like to wear in respect of European dresses like jeans, shorts fork, tops, you should choose printed material. For saris, choose the one with border and *pallau*.

For jewellery, go in for diamonds, platinum and silver, and avoid the ingrained designs. If you are wearing a *pallau*-boarder sari, then wear hanging-earrings (*jhumka*).

Although all types of skin require proper care, but dark skin needs extra care as it requires more moisture than fair skin. Dark skin develops signs of ageing rather late and dark women are luckier than the fair ones because they are less prone to pimples, shadows, wrinkles and blotches.

If you have a dark but dry skin, use a deep cleansing milk followed by a moisturiser at night. Wipe-off with a wet cotton swab, after half an hour. Take a spoonful of unboiled milk and mix a little almond oil, a few drops of lemon juice and rose water in it. Apply the mixture on your face and neck daily at night. This solution is good for clearing the complexion. Using honey is also good for glowing skin.

20. ON THE ROAD TO BEAUTY CARE

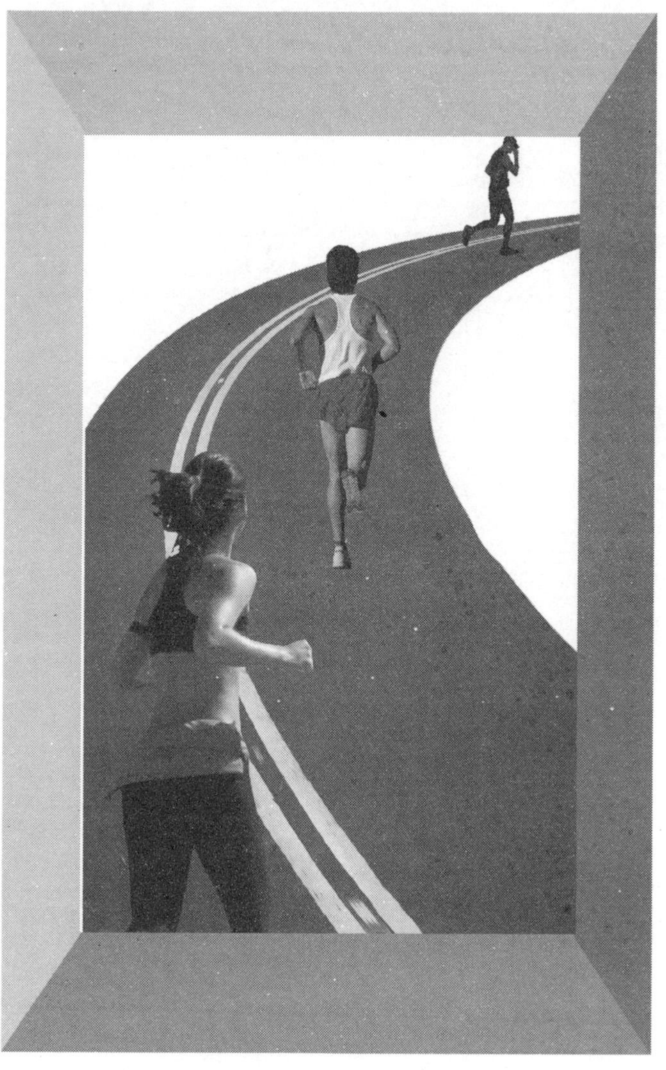

It is easier to look after ourselves when we are at home but it is tough job when we are travelling. At home, we have a set routine and we can attend to our daily personal duties with uninterrupted regularity. But, one cannot always be stationary. We may not be inveterate travellers, but, even then, we have to travel occasionally — maybe on official duty or for a visit to relatives or a pleasure trip. The routine changes and so do environment, food and climate. These changes affect the skin and looks. A beauty conscious woman needs to be alert. She should not be slack in maintaining her beauty.

While travelling, proper bathing facilities are not available and one has to adjust with make-do arrangements. Likewise, cosmetics of your choice may not be available. It is, therefore, necessary to pack the required items in your travelling kit before leaving home. You cannot carry all your cosmetics. Make a choice. Keep the non-liquid items in a plastic bag or box. Close the lid well. Pack all the things well in your vanity bag. Do not forget to carry with you your brand of talcum powder and soap. Likewise, pack your hair-oil, comb and hair-brush. Your travelling companions are — a small pair of scissors, nail-cutter, filer and scrubber. One must regularly bathe while travelling. The most worked and worn-out parts of our body during travels are our feet. Care for them well and keep them clean. Massage the soles of your feet with oil. It relieves tiredness. Keep your finger and toe-nails clean and well-trimmed. Use deep-cleansing milk every night before retiring to bed. Apply a hand lotion and body lotion on the exposed parts of your body. If you are expecting to be out in the sun the next day, better use a lacto-calamine lotion on your face.

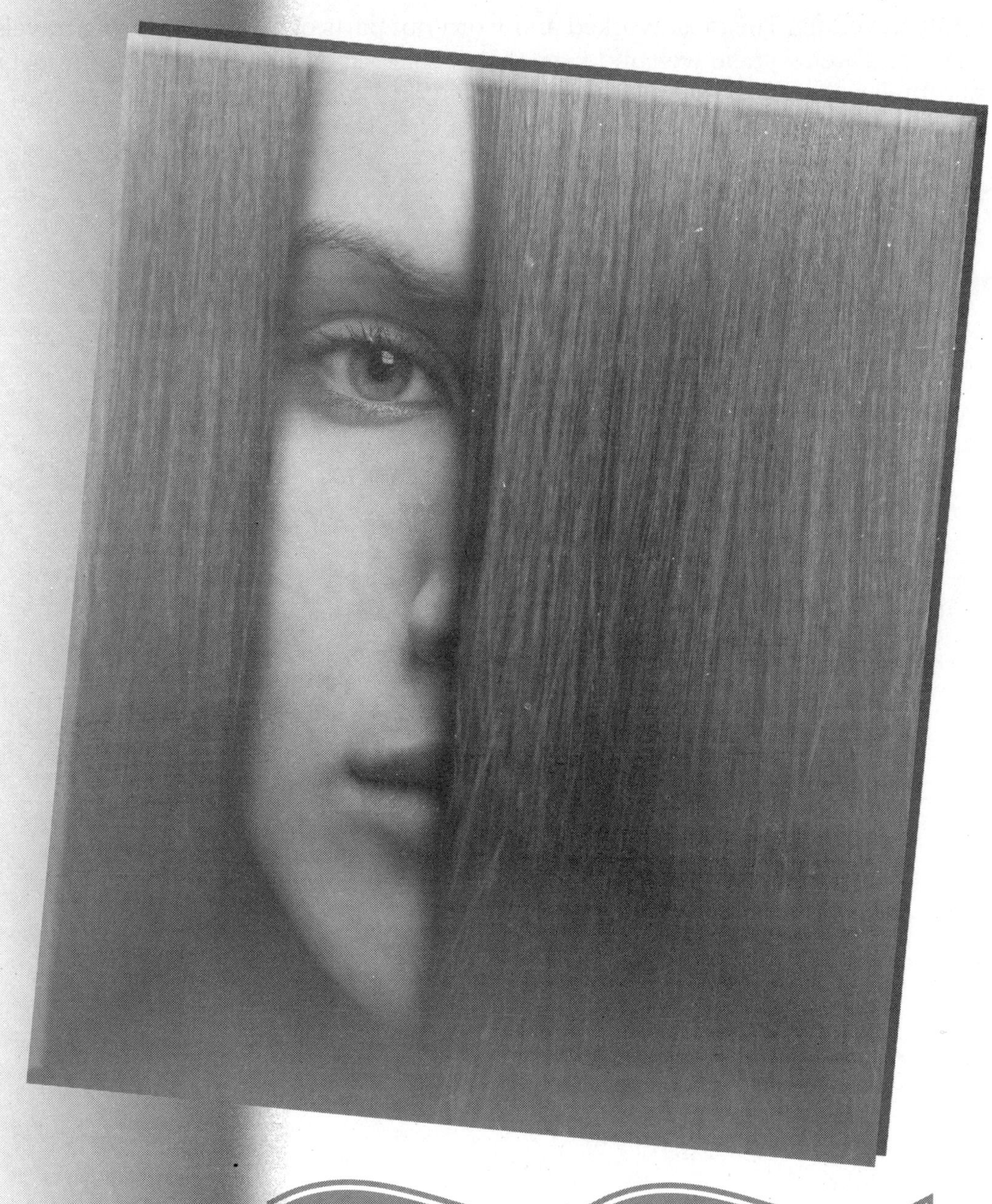

PART 3
CROWNING GLORY

21. HAIR CARE

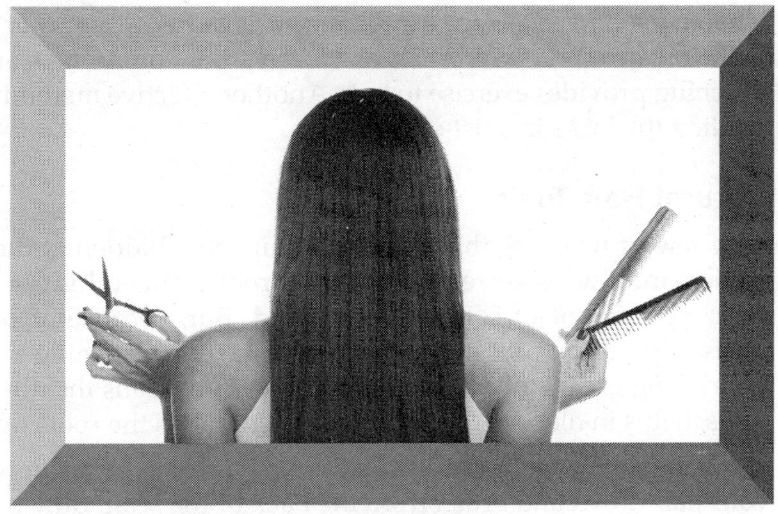

Growth of hair, its glow and health is governed by the internal system of our body. Proper care is essential for healthy hair. The skin of the scalp which is usually covered by hair, has deep-rooted hair.At the root of each hair there is a tiny bag known as papilla. Papilla provides nourishment to each hair. If one hair falls or leaves its root, papilla provides nourishment for the growth of another hair in its place. The quality of your hair depends upon your general health. Protein rich diet fruits and fresh vegetables, are good for beautiful and healthy hair. Premature greying or falling of hair signifies deficiency of nutrients in the body. Polluted atmosphere, scorching heat, sultry climate affect the beauty of hair adversely. Likewise, tension, anxiety, grief, disease, frustration, brooding are also harmful.

Hair is of 3 types — dry, oily and normal (average).

Hair Maintenance

Every hair has its own lifespan. After completing it, it falls off and a new hair sprouts in its place. The lifespan is between 2-6 years and the rate of growth is half-an-inch in 6 months. In India, hair usually remains dry because of the climate. For dry hair use, as far as possible, egg shampoo.

You can concoct a home-made solution. Take the yolk of 2 eggs, add lemon juice and rub in well on the scalp before washing. For making dry hair look shiny and healthy, take 5 spoonful of used, but dried tea leaves and 1 litre lime water. Boil the mixture, strain it when it gets cold. Apply this after shampooing and washing hair. This solution is beneficial for those who back-comb their hair. A soft massage with warm oil is also good because it activates the entire nervous system of the scalp and increases blood circulation. Before massaging, comb your hair to remove knots. Beer is good for hair. Apply it after washing hair. Beer strengthens hair roots.

Choice of Comb

Regular combing and brushing ensure healthy hair. The comb should always be clean. It should be washed in ammonia solution. Be sure that you buy a comb with rounded tips. If the ends of the comb are sharp they may injure the scalp. Comb softly and slowly to avoid damage to the roots. Plastic comb generates electricity in dry hair whereby setting becomes a problem. It is better to use a brush. Wet hair, if combed with force or jerk, will break or loosen from the roots. Comb hair 3-4 times a day. Brushing provides exercise to hair. Another effective method is to pull them slowly by holding the locks in a fist or in fingers.

Natural Hair Tonic

Very few of us know that there is a hair tonic hidden at the root of each hair. Scalp glands are always secreting oil at the roots. This oil gives gloss to the hair and an amazing amount of softness is ensured. But, because of our ignorance we let this grease dry at the root and do not let it spread. Brushing is useful in spreading this nourishing grease all over the hair. Brush also cleans the dirt and dust amassed at the roots, helps in blood circulation and strengthens the roots of the hair.

The correct method to brush your hair is to bend down from the waist, draw your hair down and brush from the back of the scalp downwards. This ensures a fast circulation of blood in the scalp. Brushing should start from the forward part, then backward part and then the sides. Slow brushing keeps the greasiness of hair intact. If already oily hair is brushed with quick movements or for longer duration, the oil glands get activated and start secreting more oil. Moreover, if you have weak, thin and very soft hair, brush slowly. If your hair is too oily, stick a piece of cotton wool or an old sock in the bristles of your brush. Extra grease will be removed.

Dry hair	**Oily hair**	**Normal hair**
➤ Shampoo once a week. ➤ Comb after drying, use hair cream or oil. ➤ Use egg shampoo.	Shampoo twice a week. Do not use oil or cream. Use lemon shampoo.	Shampoo every 10 days. Do not use extra-oily cream. Use tonic shampoo.

Dandruff

Dandruff is an enemy of the hair. It weakens the roots. Consequently, hair begins falling off. This is a kind of contagious disease. Dandruff sticks to the skin of the scalp in a cake form and blocks free flow of air to the hair roots. As a result, hair becomes weak at the roots and looses its hold. Using the comb, soap or brush of a man with dandruff should be avoided as it is contagious.

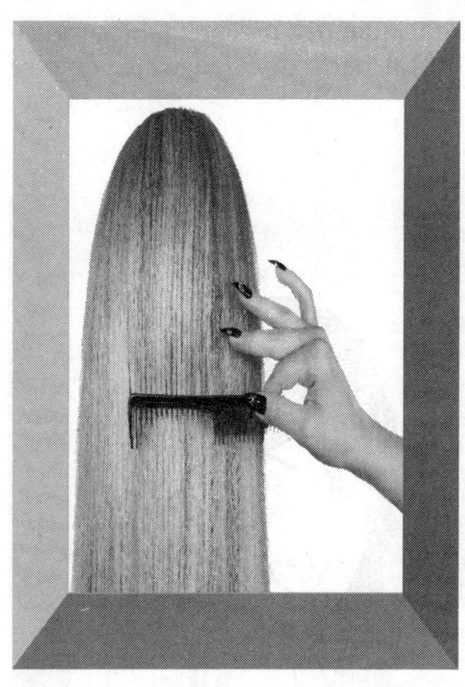

Now, an important question comes up — what is dandruff?

The cells underneath our skin are constantly undergoing changes. The dead cells fall on the skin, which are known as dandruff. If your hair is gripped by fast changes it is better to consult a doctor. Dandruff is of 2 kinds—dry and oily. Dry dandruff causes itch, while oily dandruff sticks to the scalp.

Many medicines and medicated soaps and shampoos are available to check dandruff, but the most effective is keeping your hair clean. Brush your hair at least thrice a day and shampoo once a week at least. Use of a 'pragmater ointment' at night is beneficial. While washing your hair, ensure the water does not trickle down your face. There are chances you may get pimples. Some home remedies to remove dandruff is given as follows:

- Take 6 spoonfuls of water, add 2 spoonfuls pure vinegar and apply it on the scalp with cotton wool swab before going to bed. Tie a towel around the head to protect your pillow. Wash your head next morning. After shampooing, rinse again with vinegar-water. Continue this once a week for at least three months.
- Massage the scalp with almond oil and steam-bathe your hair. Steam bathe is taken by dipping the towel in boiling water and wrapping it around the hair, like a turban. Do not let the corners of your towel be wet, so that you can hold them. When your towels gets cold repeat it 3-4 times. Steaming opens the scalp pores and increases the capacity of the hair to absorb oil from its roots (see illustration).
- You can also take a spoonful lemon juice, mix it with 2 spoonfuls vinegar and massage on the scalp. Wash your hair with an egg shampoo.

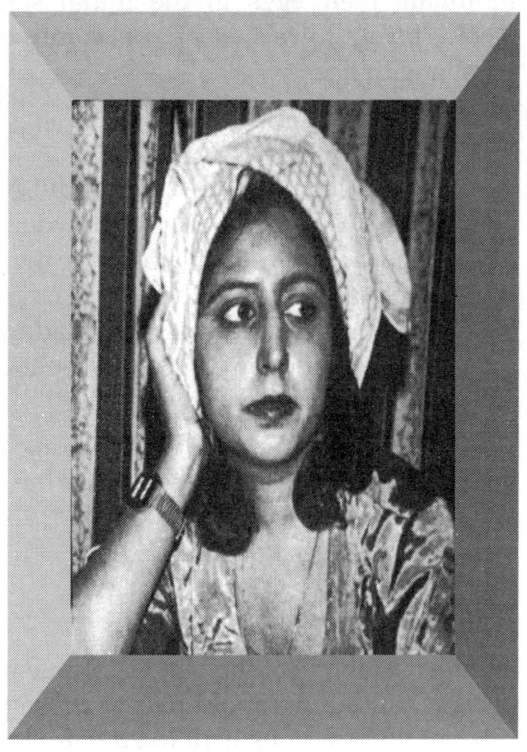

- ➤ Take 1 part almond oil, and pure sulphur in same quantity, mix and add 'surgical spirit' in equal quantitis to the above two. Put 4 parts distilled water or rose water and rub on the scalp.

Problem of Lice

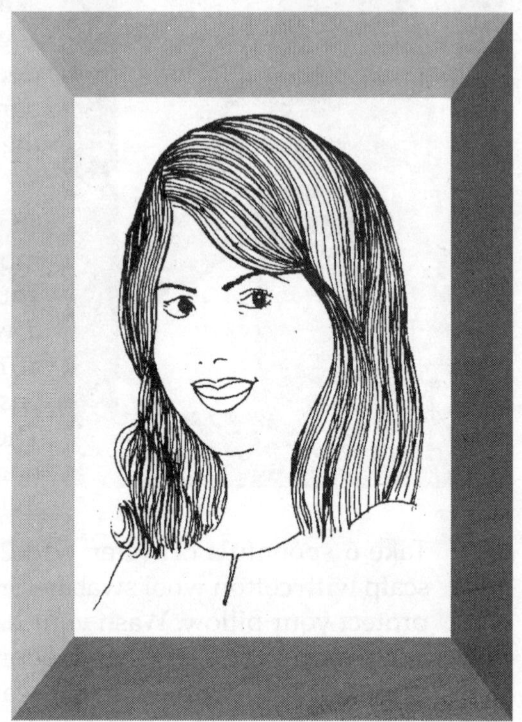

A lock of curly, black and long hair is a symbol of health and beauty. It is every woman's ardent desire to have such hair which could be the envy of others. But, hair care is a constant process and one cannot afford to be slack. Any slackness in cleanliness breeds lice. A 'louse' is a wingless parasitic insect with 6 claw-like feet. It is grey in colour but it turns brownish after sucking blood, which it does with 2 small trunk-like whiskers. A louse egg hatches in 9 days and within a fortnight the young ones attain maturity. Long hair is more prone to lice infestation.

The back portion of the head itches when infested with lice. Itch causes abrasion of the scalp skin. Lice can be controlled by removing their eggs in the initial stages. Avoid using towels, soap or comb of a person with lice.

Controlling Lice

- ➤ Take talcum powder and add 0.2 per cent 'prethrum dust' in it (or add 10 per cent DTT). Sprinkle this powder on the hair before going to bed and rub it vigorously so that it reaches the roots. Cover your mouth, nose and eyes to protect them from the powder.
- ➤ An anti-lice oil can also be made with coconut (or mustard) oil mixed with 0.2 per cent lindane (BHC) or 0.1 per cent prethrum essence. This oil can be rubbed well into the scalp to kill lice.

The above mentioned concoctions should be used at night. Tie a cloth around your head after applying any one of the medicines. Let it remain at least for 24 hours. While washing off, do not use soap or shampoo. Repeat this for a week. Lice and their eggs will both be eliminated.

Hair Fall

Falling hair is one of the biggest problems. Usually, we have hundreds and thousands of hair, and falling of old hair to make place for the new ones is a natural cycle. So, it is not quite serious if 10 to 20 hair choose to fall daily. But, when hair come out as locks and begins to thin it is a matter of concern. There are 3 stages in the process of shedding hair— normal falling, chronic baldness and temporary baldness.

Normal Fall of Hair

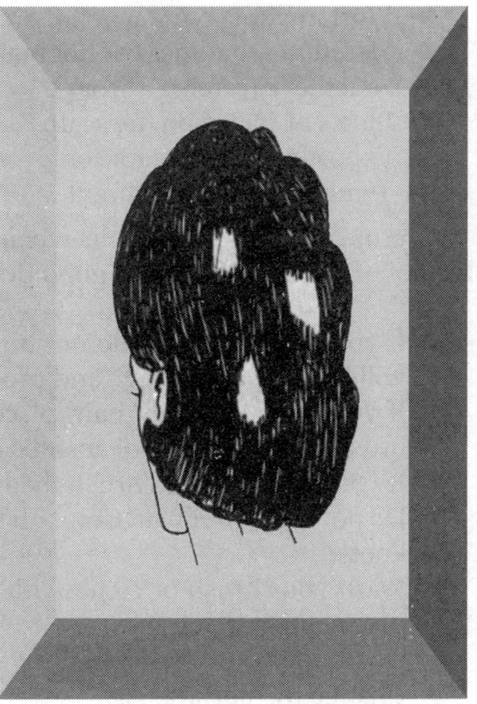

In this condition, hair fall begins gradually. Within a couple of days it becomes rapid when locks of hair start showing in the comb. This is chronic to women and can be assigned to one of the following conditions:

- Pregnancy
- Post-pregnancy
- Breast feeding
- Reaction to medicines
- High fever (typhoid, flu, malaria, etc.)

When hair begins falling suddenly without any of the above causes, try to find out the reason, and start treatment accordingly. Many a times hair fall for a while and then stops suddenly, when conditions normalize. But, if it is not controlled even after treatment, it is better to consult a doctor. Do not use too hot water for washing hair. Also ensure that you use a quality shampoo.

Temporary Baldness

Temporary baldness or 'alopecia' is on the rise among women these days. It is fall in bunches that leaves bald patches on the scalp. These patches are small in the initial stages but soon become large. Any delay in treatment results in big bald patches. But, with timely and correct treatment new hair begins to sprout. Temporary baldness is neither a skin-disease, nor contagious. The causes can be assigned to the following:

- Continuous mental tension
- Mental shock
- Anaemia or deficiency of vitamins
- Debility of the nervous system

Since the main cause of temporary baldness is mental tension, it is essential to try to banish it by creating a congenial atmosphere. In order to stabilize the nervous system, consult a good doctor. The affected area can be massaged with liquids which are helpful for blood circulation, like tincture iodine. Application of 'carbonic-snow' can also ensure blood circulation.

Permanent Baldness

Rapid hair fall is followed by baldness and if it is not treated in time, it turns into permanent baldness. Some of its causes are:

- Working or staying in a hot area
- Hereditary baldness occurring in family
- Sedentary (cerebral) work
- Burns or injury on the scalp
- Exposure to X-rays for long
- Tying hair tightly at night

Permanent baldness results when roots of hair become weak and the hair-growing faculty of the cells is dead. A good doctor should be consulted prior to treatment.

- If you have oily hair, do not brush fast or for longer time, otherwise oil glands will become over active and produce grease.
- If you have very oily hair, place a piece of cotton between the bristles of your brush. The cotton wool absorbs extra oil.
- If you have dry hair, brush them before shampooing.
- Do not brush wet hair. Comb them first with the big side of the comb and remove knots.
- Wash your brush or comb with warm soap water every week and dry them by placing up-side down
- Do not tie your hair too tightly.
- Change the parting.
- Protect yourself from bright sun, moisture, mental excitement, worries and frustrations. These are detrimental to beautiful, healthy hair.

22. CHOOSING THE RIGHT SHAMPOO

A well set hair encompasses healthy, clean and lustrous hair. For cleanliness, regular washing of hair is essential. Apart from the traditional methods, shampoo is the best method. Soap is harmful for hair and so are sub-standard products. While washing your hair shampoo should be used properly. Do not simply empty the contents directly from the bottle on the head and wash off the lather. This way the nourishing chemicals do not get a chance to reach the roots and a large part of the shampoo is wasted. It is, therefore, important to know how to use shampoo effectively.

Selecting Shampoo

The market is flooded with large varities of shampoos of different brands, but it is safer to be selection and buy only products of well-known companies. Sub-standard products may be cheaper, but they are harmful. Moreover, buy from shops to safeguard against imitations.

Shampoos have different compositions — without soap, with egg, with conditioner and so on. Soapless shampoo contains chemicals which remove dirt and leave the hair clean and lustrous. For dry hair, egg shampoo is beneficial; for oily hair, lemon shampoo, and for normal hair tonic shampoo should be used. If you have the problem of falling hair, consult a specialist and use medicated shampoo, as per his advice.

Although a large number of products are available in the market shampoos can be prepared at home as well, you will get a pure product at nominal cost. A couple of recipes for and thereby making shampoo at home are as follows:

- Take bar of soap nuts (*reetha*), dry *amla* and *shikakai* in a quantity of 50 gram each. Grind them to a fine powder. Boil the powder for half an hour in 2 litres of water. Strain it when it gets cold, and fill it in a bottle.
- For dyed hair, make egg shampoo. Take the yolk (yellow part) of 20 two eggs, beat it and mix a little water in it. Now, beat the white part and mix it with the beaten yolk. Wet your hair with lukewarm water and apply the shampoo. Wash your hair again with luke-warm water and apply the remaining shampoo.

Dry Shampoo

Dry shampoo is a powder containing chemicals and mineral salts. For cleaning hair you need not wet them, nor wash them. Just sprinkle the powder and comb or brush. Hair will be clean. Dry shampoo is not easily available in our country.

Dye Shampoo

This product dyes the hair while it cleans. It is available in different shades. The hair is dyed according to the shade you are using. These are temporary dyes. Since these dyes are chemically prepared, they may adversely affect the hair. Pregnant women and those suffering from skin-diseases should not use dye shampoo. It should not be used during menstruation period. Dye shampoo, too, is not very popular in our country.

Correct Use of Shampoo

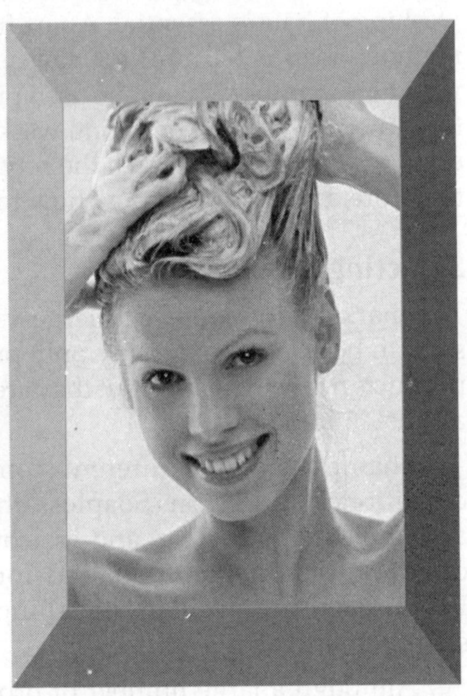

Shampoo your hair once a week in summer. If you have oily hair, shampoo twice a week. In winter, shampoo should be done once in 10-12 days. If you have dry hair, you can shampoo once a fortnight. Before washing, massage oil into the scalp for 10-15 minutes. Do not wash immediately after massage because massage stimulates the blood vessels, increases blood circulation and warms up the area. So, better wait for an hour or so. For extreme dry hair, massage with warm olive oil.

Do not use large quantities of shampoo in one go. It will go waste. Wet your hair, take a spoonful on your left palm and rub well all over the scalp with your right hand. Let it soak into the skin, produce foam and wash off. Apply it again similarly and wash off. Now, wash your head well with plenty of water.

Hair Conditioner

Apply hair conditioner when the hair is dry. Conditioner is identical to shampoo. It is easily available. Rub it into the scalp gently for a couple of minutes so that it reaches the roots and gets absorbed. Wash hair again but do not scrub too hard or use too much water. Otherwise, it will wash off. Conditioner gives a security cover to the hair and makes them lustre. Hair can be dried either by wrapping a towel around the head or with the help of a hair-dryer.

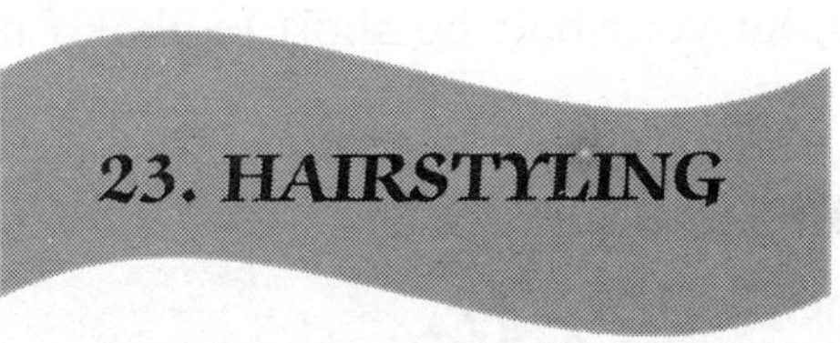

23. HAIRSTYLING

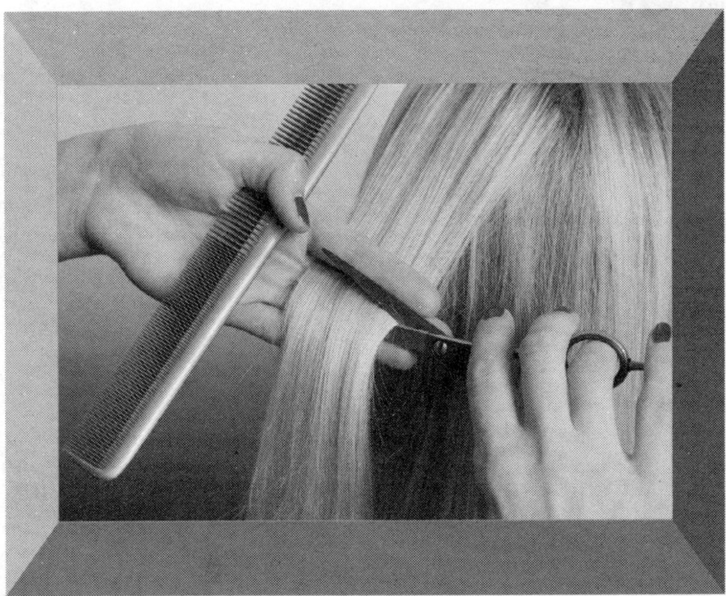

To a large extent a woman's beauty depends on her hairstyle. A woman's charm is enhanced if her hair is set according to the face and body. Face can be round, flat, oval and oblong. Hair should be styled according to the shape of the face. You are the best judge to decide which style suits you. Look at the a mirror and decide. If you are unable to decide, take the help of a beautician. Here are some hints for you to choose the right-style:

Round Face

Straight and untied hair make a round face look longish and attractive. The end of the hair should be as long as the end of the chin.

Oblong Face

For a long face, short hair spread at the end on the sides look attractive. Longish style does not suit a long face.

Oval Face

An oval face usually has a broad forehead and a pointed chin. Hair should be spread at the top and clinging at the bottom so that the face appears symmetrical. Do not part hair in the middle.

Flat Face

Curls look attractive on a flat face. Let hair dangle on the forehead, eyes and temples so that they appear scattered. Do not part your hair in the middle.

Short Neck

If you have a short neck, let your hair be short so that a major part of the neck is exposed.

Small Forehead and Broad Jaw

Hair should be trimmed at the front. Back combing is advisable. For a broad jaw have a hair-cut which comes upto the jaws so that the breadth is hidden and jaws looks small.

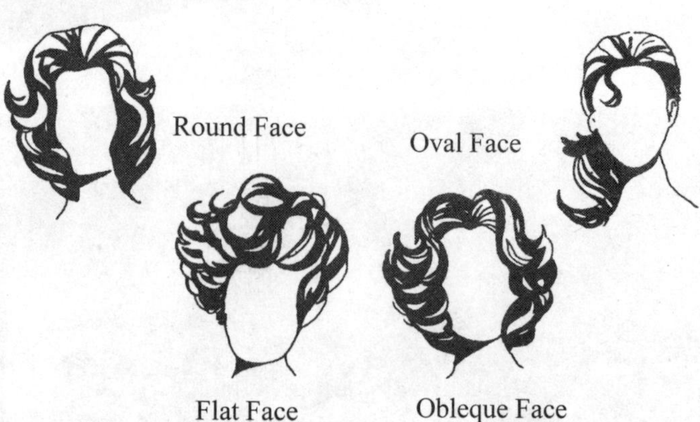

Small Chin

For a small chin, go for a hair-cut that reaches the chin and roll the ends inwards so that the ears and chin are partly covered.

Large Ears

If ears are proportionately large, try to hide them. Have a hair-cut on the sides with ends rolled inward towards the ears.

Tall Height, Slim Body

Any hair-style suits this figure. Shoulder cuts look particularly attractive.

Tall Height, Fat Body

An obese body looks unattractive with too short or too long hair. Short hair on a fat person make her appear too short and fat.

Short Height, Slim Body

Any style will suit but do not go for very long hair. Scattered hair make the upper part look obese.

Short Height, Fat Body

Have a cut only upto jaws. Do not scatter the hair. The body will look fat.

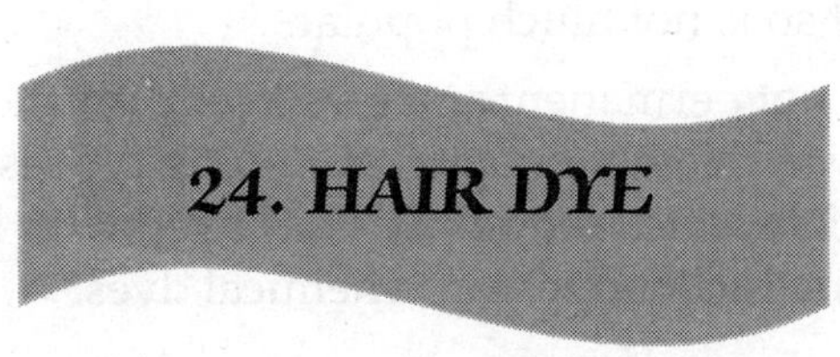

24. HAIR DYE

There was a time when grey hair was symbolic of old age and was looked upon with reverence. It signified seniority and experience. But, things have changed now. Most young men's and women's hair are going pre-maturly grey, and hence they are left with no option but to resort to dying. In European and other Western countries hair dying is a fashion. Women bleach their hair and dye in different colours. In our country, however, hair dying is a necessity for most women. Indian women prefer only natural shades—black or dark brown.

With advancing age, greying starts with random grey hair but soon it catches on rapidly. On spotting 1 or 2 grey hair, women tend to pull them out, which is a wrong practice. One hair so pulled gives birth to a couple of other grey hair. When hair is pulled with a jerk, the root secretes a liquid which spreads to the other hair affecting them too. They also turn grey. If at all you wish to get rid of the few grey hair you have, do not pull them. Clip them off with small scissors near the root. Many a times, grey hair loosen all by themselves and come off while brushing or combing.

How to Dye

Dyeing is an art and has to be done with care. Only using a dye is not enough, using it skillfully is necessary to make them look natural and attractive. Hair can be dyed by 3 methods:

(i) Dyeing with dye shampoo or colouring oil.
(ii) Dyeing with herbs.
(iii) Dyeing with chemical dyes. In India we do not use dye shampoo or oil. We depend much on herbal dyes and chemical dyes.

Herbal Dyes

Herbal dyes are not permanent. Moreover, it is a slow process, and must be continued for long. Herbs used for dyeing are—henna, walnut bark and tea-leaves. Of these, henna (*mehandi*) is more popular, though it gives a reddish-brown tinge. *Mehandi* leaves are ground to a powder. Adding water, make a paste. Apply it, let it dry and wash with cold water. *Mehandi* is to be used twice since one application as it does not give colour in the first attempt.

Walnut bark : Soak it into water for 12 hours approximately, strain it and put a little ammonia. This dye gives a light brown tinge.

Tea Leaves : Boil well in water till it leaves its colour. Let it cool. Apply on hair. This is not a permanent dye and so is not much popular.

Since herbal dyes are not permanent and give a reddish and light brown tinge, they are less in vogue. Moreover, dyeing with herbs is a long process and has to be repeated for months together to achieve desired result. Hair dyed with herbs are difficult to set. People, therefore, are more inclined toward chemical dyes.

Chemical Dyes

This is a popular dyeing method in our country. The dye is more or less permanent and if dyed well, hair look almost black. The dye is not affected by climate, season, water and soap. These dyes are made with chemicals like 'para', hydrogen peroxide and others, and are easily available in the market.

For dyeing, wash your hair clean, remove all grease and apply the dye as per instructions, with a brush. Dye leaves colour on the fingers and nails so, use rubber gloves. Do not apply the dye on the skin of your scalp, apply on hair only. Leave the on dye for one hour and wash it off with shampoo. Dye after a fortnight or so, because when hair grows, roots begin to show grey.

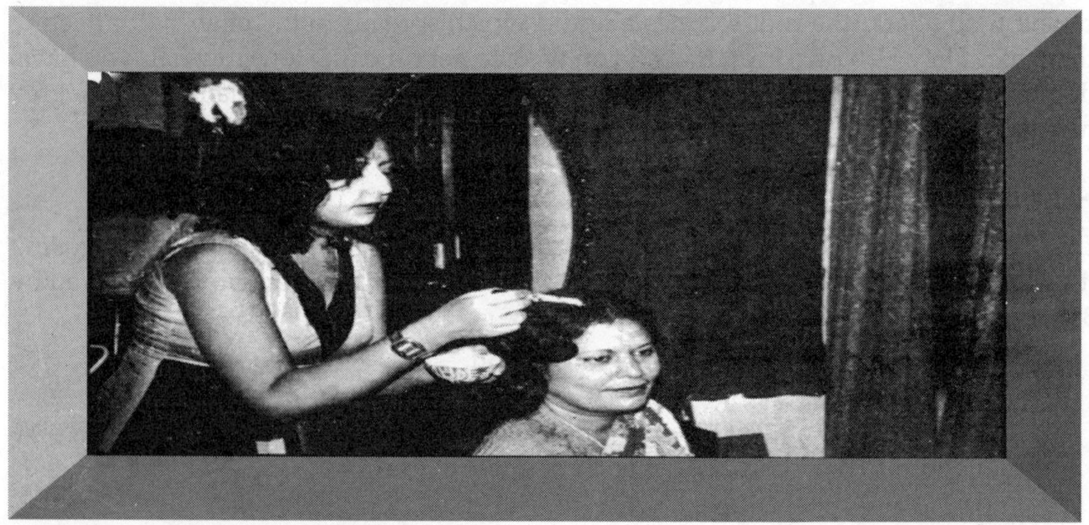

Ill-effects of Chemical Dyes

The chemicals used in dyes cause reaction on the skin. In many cases, the burning sensation does not start immediately after dyeing but can take 48 hours to occur. Reddishness shows in the ears, spreads to the eyes and then to the whole face. Some may even get eczema. It is, therefore, advisable to take a 'skin-test' by applying some dye behind the ears or on the neck. Let it dry and apply again. This test can be done on the inner part of the elbow where the skin is tender. If there is no reaction within 48 hours, go ahead and dye. But, there is no guarantee that you are immune to reaction for ever. It is better to test every time before dye is used.

In case of reaction on the skin, consult a doctor and take prescribed medicine. In order to ward off the ill-effects of 'para' chemical, use water with sodium chloride to clean your hair. This mixture is made thus: 2 litres water, 2 table spoonfuls of sodium chloride, 1 table spoonful hydrogen peroxide. Mix these and wash hair with the mixture twice a day. It is, however, necessary to consult a doctor in case of any skin abrasion or reaction. If a doctor is not available, take one of the following solutions and apply it on skin with a hanky:

- Take fresh, clean water. Add boric powder and apply on the affected part.
- Take 10 'camomile' flower, put them in boiling water. Strain the mixture and apply when it gets cold.

Do not dye in case the following conditions prevail:

- During menstruation period
- During pregnancy
- After child birth till the child is suckling
- If you are suffering from any skin-disease
- In case of asthma, heart trouble or kidney problem
- If you feel burning sensation while dyeing
- If you have falling hair.
- If hair is extremely dry

***

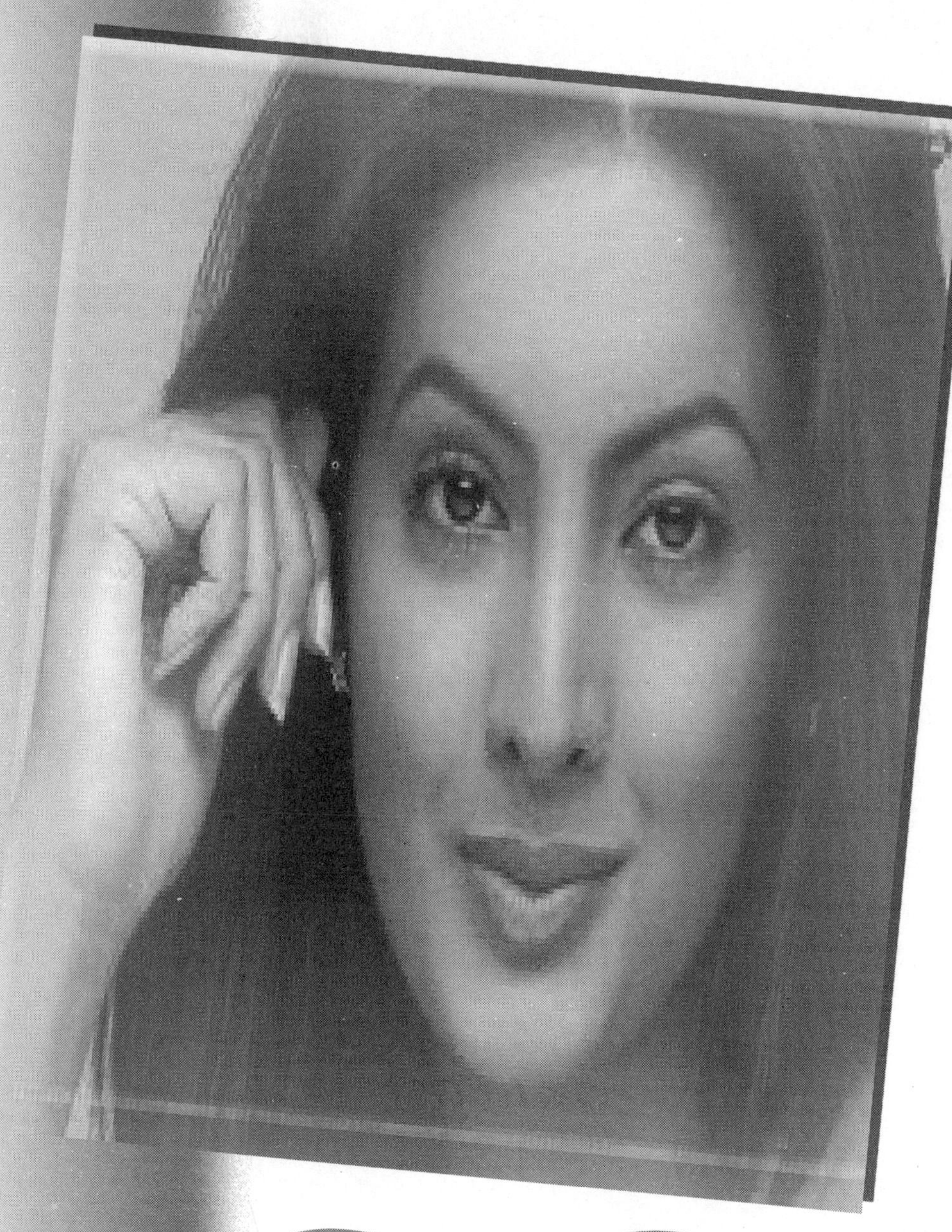

PART 4
BEAUTIFUL BODY

25. BEAUTY OF A SWAN NECK

Massage and exercise can make a short or thick neck shapely and beautiful. Massage daily for 15-20 minutes either with lukewarm olive oil or mustard oil. Start with the back of the neck (as illustrated in Figure 1), massaging with both hands from the upper to the lower part. Then massage right and left parts of the neck. Now, reverse the process and massage from the lower part of the neck to the upper part (as illustrated in Figure 2). In winter, massage with nourishing or cold cream mixed with a little almond oil.

Some of the exercises given here are useful for a long, shapely neck.

Stand straight. Move your neck once to the right and once to the left and try to touch your shoulder with the chin (as illustrated in Figure 3). Keep your head straight and bend it slowly forward till the chin touches the chest. Raise it slowly and take it backwards till it touches the inward part of the shoulders (see Figure 4). Repeat these exercises 20-25 times.

Lie down on the bed with your head dangling down, raise it slowly while lying down. It stretches the neck.

Usually, neck is a neglected part of the body. But, a clean and healthy neck is as much important for an attractive personality, as a healthy, charming face. While taking bath, the neck should be scrubbed well with soap. Sometimes neck looks darker than the face. It is, therefore, necessary to apply make-up on the neck also along with the face to ensure that both look alike in complexion. Before retiring to bed, the neck should also be cleaned with a cleansing milk-cream. Wash it with tepid water, apply glycerine and dab with a soft towel to prevent wrinkles. Also apply a face-pack once a week on the neck to ensure its softness. You can use a paste made with one spoonful of gram flour (besan) and one spoonful of curd; apply it on the neck leaving it there for 15-20 minutes. If the neck is dark, it can be bleached once a fortnight.

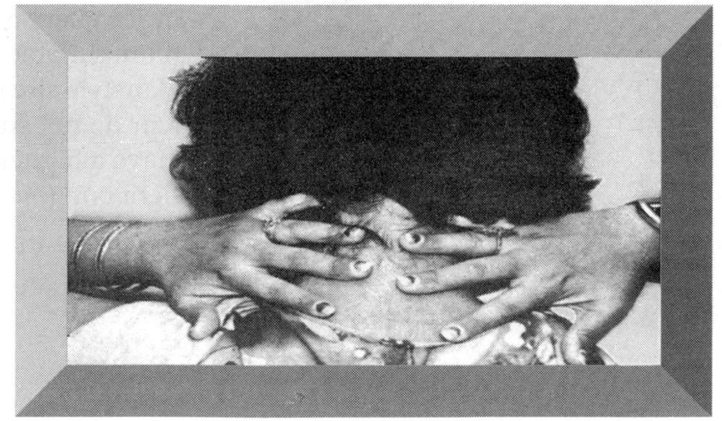

1

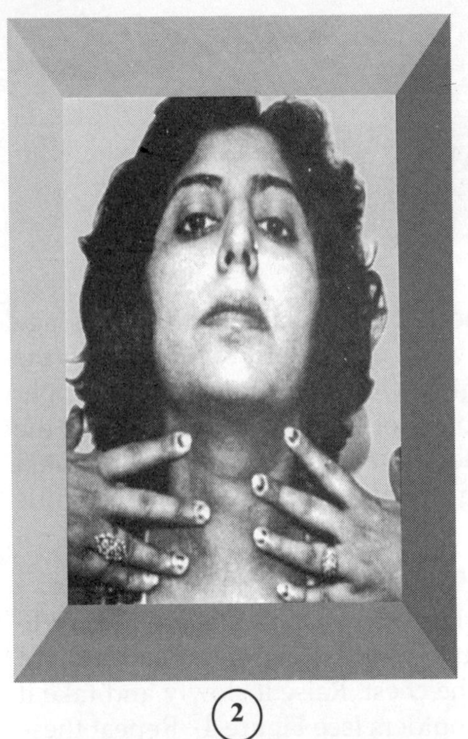

2

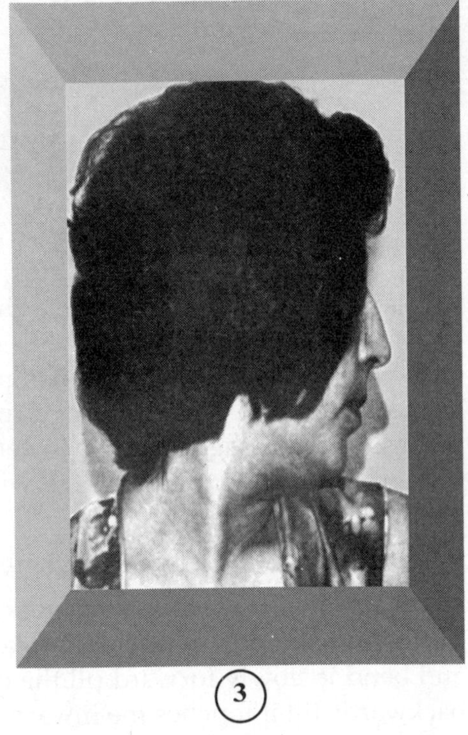

3

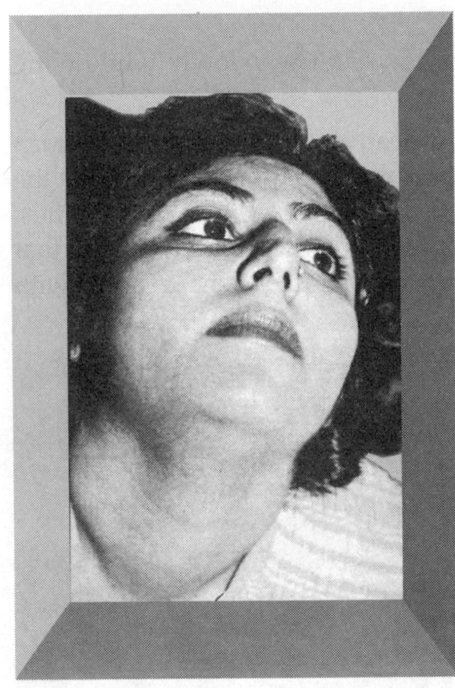

4

Tips

- If you have a short neck, do not wear a high-neck blouse or shirt.
- Use 'V'- shape or low-neck dresses to give your neck a longish look.
- A short neck does not look beautiful with jewellery or big ear-rings. Simple designs in jewellery, small eartops or earrings are more suitable.
- Hairstyle also matters. Dishevelled, scattered hair do not suit a person with a short neck. Have a higher hair-style like pony-tale or a tight bun (*juda*).

***

26. FIXING A DOUBLE CHIN

Obesity shows itself as much on your face and chin as on other parts of the body. Usually, the chin becomes flabby and appears 'double', which is called 'double chin'. Although 'double chin' is a common factor for both men and women, it is rather unwelcome in case of women because it mars their looks. Regular exercise and dieting may reduce weight but leave behind the flabbiness. Flabbiness below the chin becomes a problem.

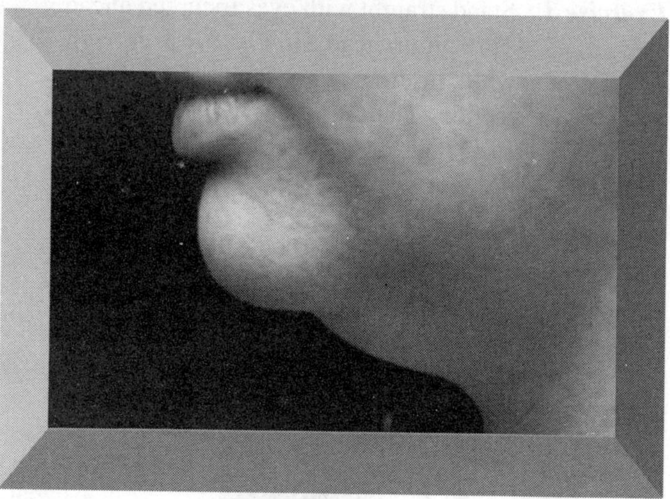

Diet and Massage

Take a light, balanced and nourishing diet. Eat a little less than your appetite. A normal healthy person requires 1300 to 1600 calories in 24 hours. Avoid fried and greasy food; instead increase the intake of milk, cheese, seasonal fruits and green vegetables. These strengthen the muscles.

Regular massage helps reduce flabbiness of chin. It tightens the muscles. The best time to massage is half an hour before taking bath. But before massaging, remove all traces of make-up, otherwise they clog the pores, making massaging ineffective. For a good massage, use cream. Apply it on the chin and rub gently from the neck above, towards the chin. Do not massage from up to down because this process wrinkles the skin. After massage, stroke the flabby part gently with fingers. Now, hold the 'double chin' between a pinch of your forefinger and thumb and stretch it left and right (see illustration). Lastly, massage slowly stretching the flabby part towards your temples.

Exercises

Here are some effective exercises to prevent a 'double-chin':

Exercise 1 : Sit erect, take your head backwards as far as you can, then come to the original position. Repeat it 5 times. Increase it once a day till 10.

Exercise 2 : Sit in a chair with a table in front, placing your elbows on the table. Now put your face between your palms and stroke your chin gently (10 times) with the end of your palms. Do not stroke too hard.

Exercise 3 : Stand straight with eyes focussed ahead. Turn your head slowly towards right while turning your eyes in the same direction. Then repeat it towards the left. Repeat several times.

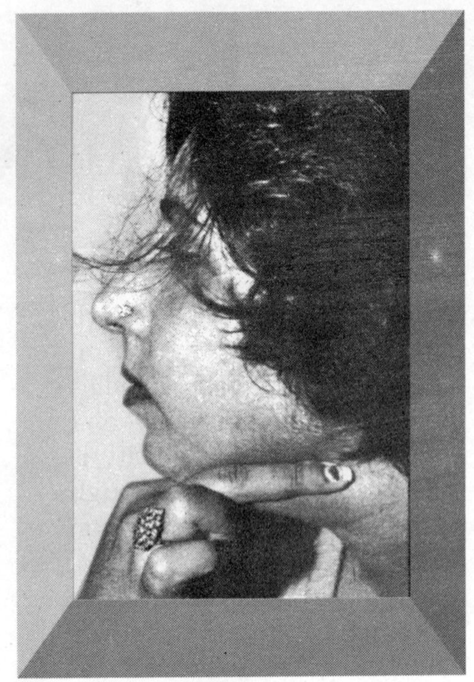

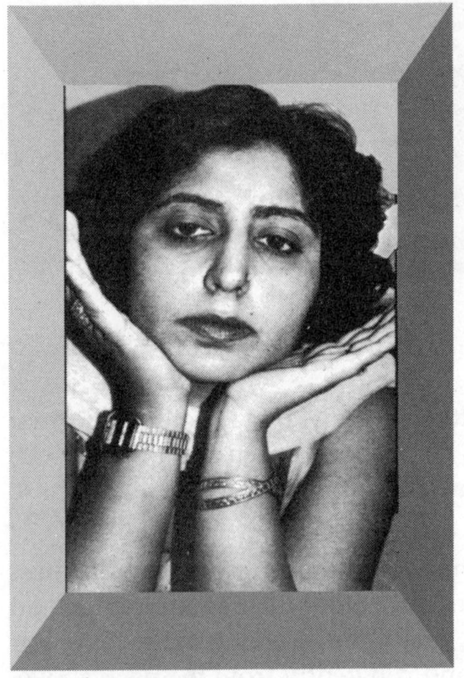

Exercise 4 : Sit erect on the floor and bend your head backward so that the flabby fat below your chin gets stretched. Now, bend backward fully and touch the ground with your head taking care that your heels are placed firmly on the ground. Inhale and lift your head slowly. Exhale and lift your body.

Calltion : Women with 'double chin' should not use pillow while sleeping.

***

27. BEAUTIFUL BOSOM

A full basom and altractive and breastline is a symbol of feminine beauty. A female becomes aware of her breasts as soon as she steps out of her adolescence and attains youth. Although shapely breasts are the gift of nature, their maintenance is in your own hands. Timely care since early adolescence, when a woman is in her formative years, can help her in keeping the breastline attractive. A girl goes through rapid body changes between 12-14 years of age when her breasts begain to develop. Between 14-18 they develop fully. However, sometimes growth is stunted due to hormonal imbalance, congenital defects or deficiency of nourishing diet. Wearing good brassieres during the developmental years is advisable to prevent sagging in the later years. But, brassieres should not be worn too tight. It may be one of the causes of cancer eventually. During developmental period girls should go in for activities like swimming, skipping, badminton, table-tennis, swinging, riding which give vigorous exercise to the upper portion of the body.

Breasts begain to sag and lose their tautness after delivery, or during long illness, pregnancy or because of irregular menstruation. These women require a balanced diet. Inclusion of protein, carbohydrates, fats, vitamins, calcium, salts and minerals in sufficient quantities is essential. The best way to maintain your breast is to massage with olive daily before bath. Massage should be done in circular movements from the lower part of the breasts to the upper. A cold water bath thereafter ensures rapid blood circulation and growth.

Breasts require maximum attention Post Child birth. Since it is not advisable to do heavy exercises, one should start doing light ones like 'palm pressing'. Kneel down and press your palms in 'namaskar' pose in the centre of the chest so that the tissues around the breasts are under full pressure. Exhale slowly and release the pressure. Repeat 10-15 times a day. Another light exercise is spread both hands and place your palms on a wall in front of you. Press your palms and you will feel pressure on your veins and tissues as a result they will stretch (See Figure 1).

Likewise breast-feeding mothers also have to take extra care. Breasts sag if the infant is suckled while sitting or reclining in a faulty posture. For example, suckling with the infant on the lap or suckling lying down is harmful for the breasts. Always suckle in a sitting position with the child on the lap and your hand under its head so as to lift it and keep its head steady. Press the nipples immediately after suckling and remove the remaining milk with a couple of jerks. This gives lightness and freshness to the breasts. Bathe the breasts with hot and cold baths simultaneously to ensure rapid blood circulation. Sprinkle hot water and then cold, 4-5 times alternately.

An easy exercise for sturdy breasts is as follows: Stand straight with arms dangling on your sides. Raise each arm above the heads and turn round alternately. Repeat 10-15 times.

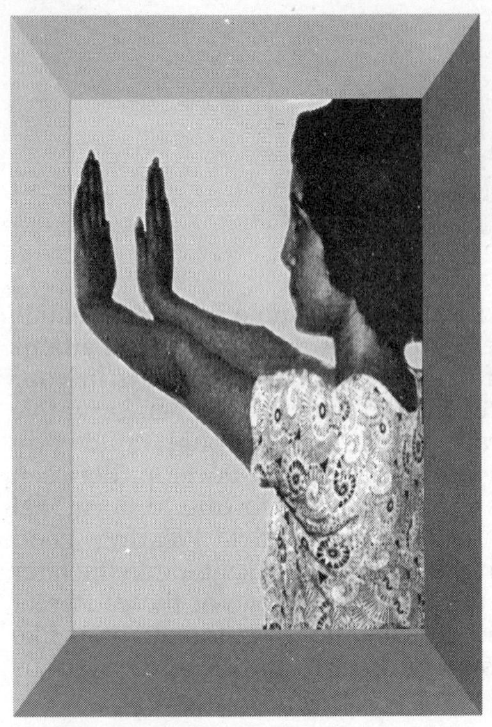

Usually I get clients in my clinic with breast problems. Some have under-developed breasts while some have too large breasts. Those with small breasts use heavily padded bras without realising that the thick, synthetic (or nylon) padded brassieres heat the glands and may eventually result in cancerous growth. Likewise very tight bras are also damaging. It is essential to remove your bra at night. Many married women have a peculiar problem with one breast being smaller than the other. It is because of the suckling of the child more on one side than the other. Even some unmarried women develop this problem. However, this is not a matter of concern. If you have small breasts, massage them with a nourishing cream. You can also exercise. One of them is as follows: The arm on the side of the small breast should be spread in front and then move it round 10-15 times, first clockwise then anti-clockwise.

I also get clients with very heavy breasts. They dangle because of overweight and pain slightly. In Western countries, extra flesh is removed surgically. This is an expensive proposition and is beyond our means. Various creams and lotions and pills are available these days to make breasts smaller or larger, but it is wise to avoid them. You can at best choose your bras wisely. For large breasts use a soft round cupped brassiere. Avoid low cut blouses.

Yogasana for Beauty of Breasts

Bhujangasana is useful for a proper breast development. Lie down on your stomach, place palms on the ground in front of you and lift up the fore-part of the body so that the muscles are stretched (see illustration).

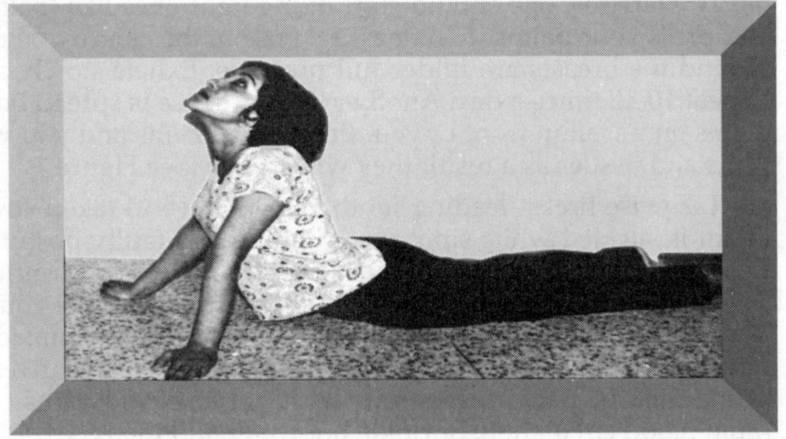

***

28. BEAUTIFUL AND SHAPELY BACK

Usually, women take extra care to beautify their face with make-up and cosmetics, but a glance at their back proves disappointing. Since the back is exposed in most-cases because of the outfit — low-neck and short blouses — it is essential to take care of it. Agreed that scrubbing and cleaning the back is not easy which results in accumulation of layers of dirt on the back, but some measures are to be evolved to clean it. Particularly women with oily skin suffer more because the skin gets black patches and rashes due to dirt. This part becomes itchy and when scratched irritation increases and rashes spread, leaving permanent marks. Those suffering from dandruff in the hair, get it on the back also. It leaves blotches and since the area cannot be reached easily for cleaning, the entire back becomes dark.

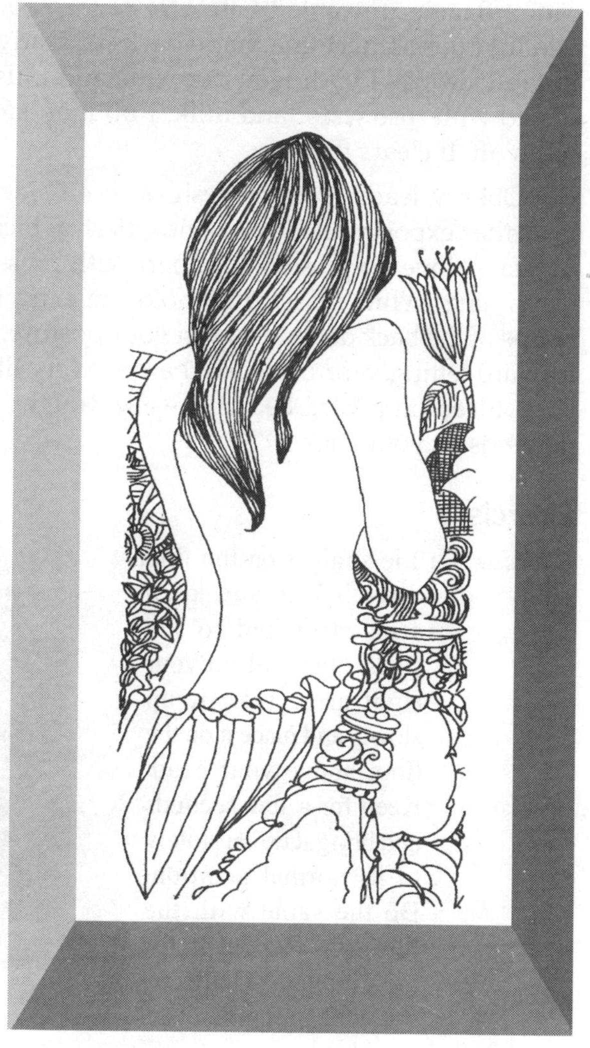

Apart from this, other sore points are flabbiness due to general obesity and the growth of hair on the back. To counter these, effective measures, like massage, packs, bleaching, dieting and exercises can be taken.

Treatment

To heal rashes due to dandruff, use medicated soap for bathing. Also be careful while washing your hair so that the water containing dandruff does not trickle down the back. This is a precaution to counter the contagious attack of dandruff. Rub in some acne lotion at night and wear something loose to avoid itching. Before bath, massage with mustard oil, wait for 5-10 minutes and then scrub well. It will remove dirt. If soap is not effective to clean the back, make a paste with milk and maida, coat it on the back, leave for 10 minutes and wash off with warm water. This clears the skin of its darkness or of its bronze shade acquired due to exposure. Lemon is also effective. Cut a lemon into small pieces and rub them on the back. Let the juice dry. It will take 10 minutes. Wash off with cold water.

Some women have hair-growth on their back. These can be hidden by bleaching. Wash off with hot water, apply cold cream thereafter. This can be repeated twice a month. It will remove the dark patches and give a shine to the back by concealing or camouflaging unwanted hair. Use of face-pack on the back ensures a beautiful, soft and lustrous skin. Home-made packs or ready-made packs can prove more beneficial, if a few drops of hydrogen peroxide and mustard oil are mixed in it. Also, try besan mixed with rose water and milk. Rub it on face, neck and back. Let it dry for a while, wash off. It clears the skin.

Obesity leads to extra flesh on both sides of your spine. Fitting blouses tighten it further exposing flabby sagging flesh which looks ugly. This can be removed by a massage done by pressing the part with pressure. Balanced diet is also effective, so is swimming. While massaging, hold the extra flesh in a pinch and move it vigorously. Shape of the back depends upon your posture. If you leave it loose while sitting or bend forward letting your back lax, there is every likelihood that you may develop a hunch-back. Sleep on a hard bed and walk straight. Much of the appeal of your personality depends on your back.

Exercises

Exercise 1 : Lie straight on the floor. Stretch legs and keep arms stretched to the sides. Now, lift up your right arm. Take it up slowly and place it on the floor above your head. Keep for a few seconds and bring it down slowly to its normal position. Do the same with the left arm. Repeat it for three minutes. This exercise will strengthen back muscles.

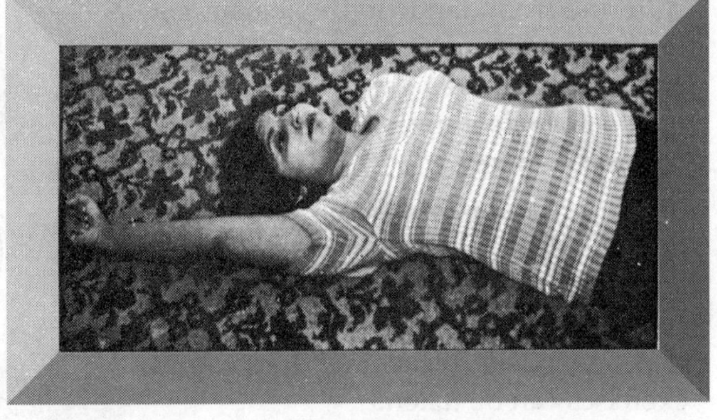

Exercise 2 : Sit on the floor on your knees like for *namaz*. Stretch your arms straight above your head. Bend down slowly and touch the floor with your fingers. Repeat daily for 10-15 times.

Exercise 3: Lie down straight on the floor, stretch your arms straight, placing them near the sides of the knees. Lift your back as much as you can without moving your head, arms or legs. Repeat 10 times.

Exercise 4 : Sit straight on a plank *(chawki),* stretch legs straight. Stretch arms above your head and start bending forward slowly making a 45 degree angle. Without changing your position, try to take back your arms. Come into original position. Repeat 5-10 times.

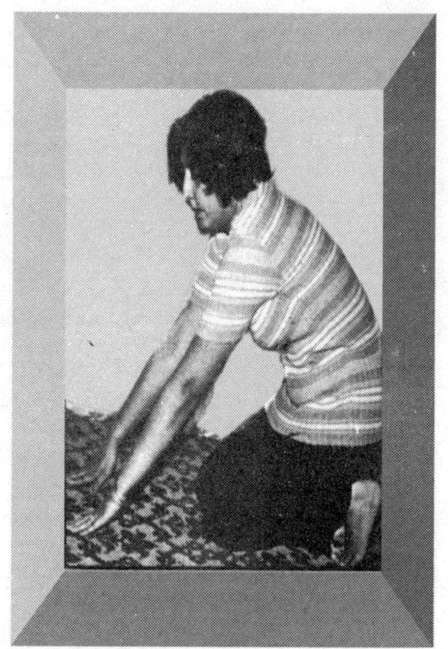

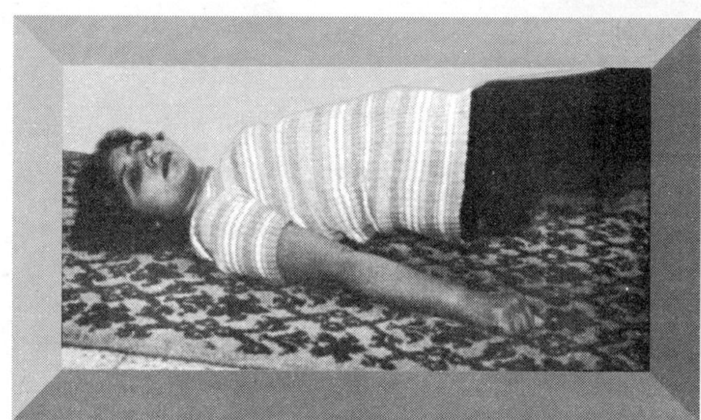

Note : Exercises should be done in the morning before bathing and on an empty stomach.

To ascertain an even complexion use foundation on your back along with face and neck. Also use compact powder.

29. GET THE PERFECT WAISTLINE

A slim waistline between shapely hips and prominent breasts makes a woman highly appealling. This lends flexibility to her frame and grace to her gait. Hip-bone of women is broader than of men. After child-birth, in particular, one develops fattening tendency and the waist becomes flabby losing its natural beauty.

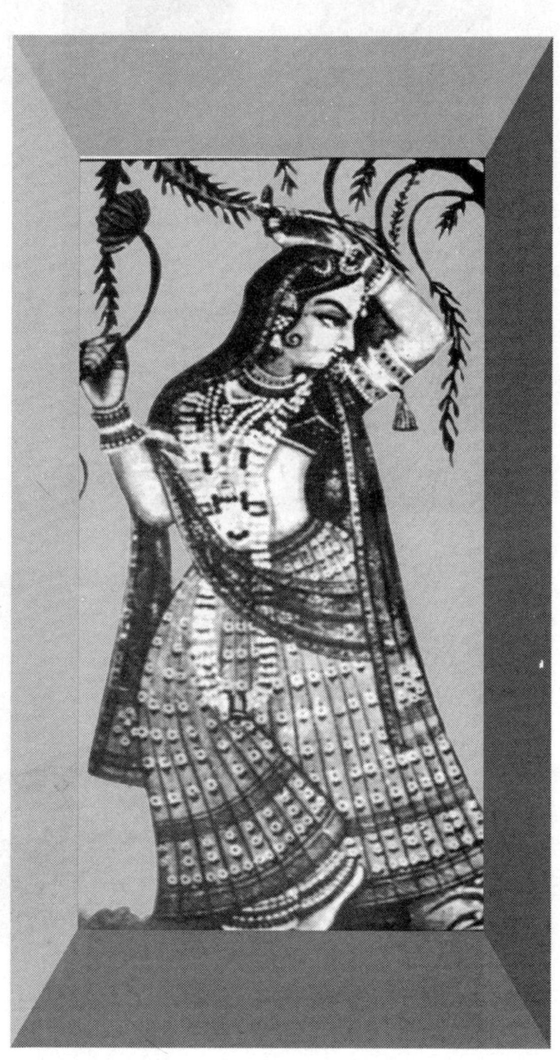

Suggestions

Avoiding fried and greasy food and regular massaging with olive oil are important to maintain slim and trim waistline. Likewise, regular exerciseis also helpful in maintaining it. Morning walks, rope jumping, grinding (*chakki* of days of yore), dance, drawing well-water, swimming provide natural exercises. Here are some suggestions for a beautiful, shapely and flexible waist:

- During pregnancy and after delivery, take care to massage regularly with olive oil to prevent wrinkles, flabbiness and folds.
- Do not use a high pillow. It deforms and weakens waist.
- Hard bed is good for maintaining a straight back whereas soft bed or foam mattresses bend it.
- These days attractive advertisements claim to restore your slim waistline by the use of belts or corsets. But, their use is medically not advisable. These gadgets do ensure tightness, but they hinder the blood circulation and leave ill-effects on the body, particularly on the uterus, which may give rise to many problems.

Few exercises for waist are given below:

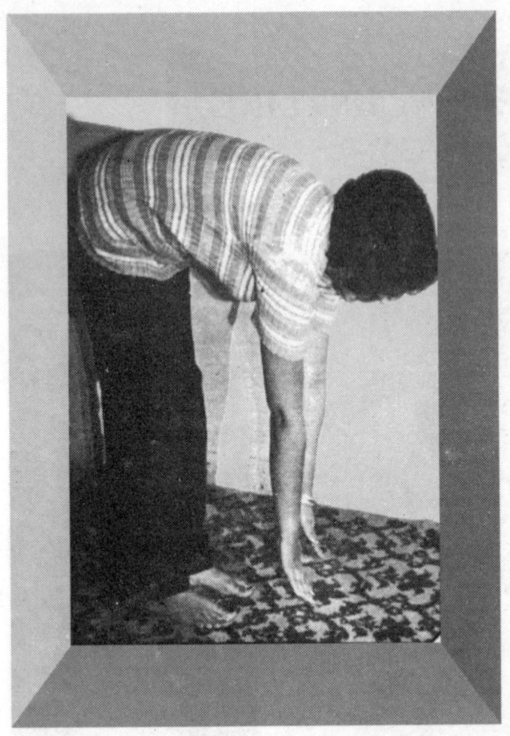

1. Stand erect, joining both feet. Bend down and touch your toes, keep legs straight at knees. Repeat it 10-15 times.

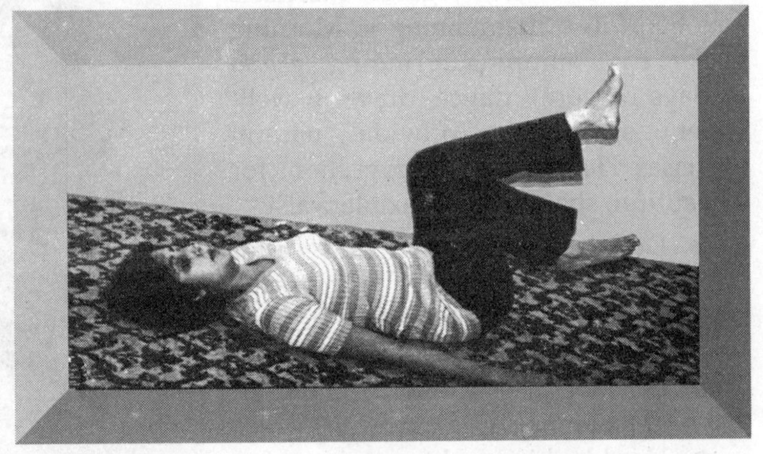

2. Lie down on your back and move legs like cycling.

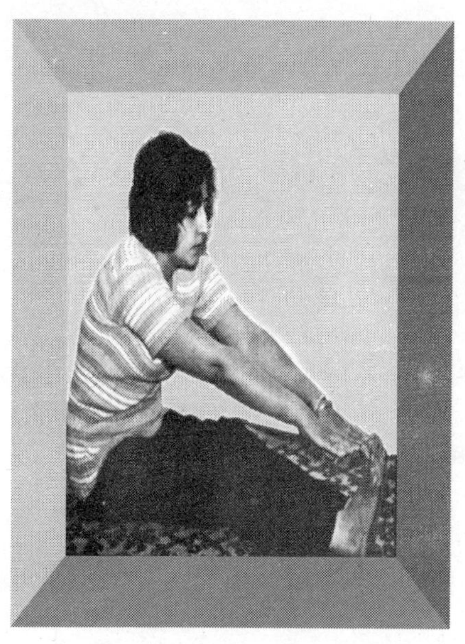

3. Sit on ground with legs stretched in front. Try to touch toes, do not bend knees. Repeat 10 times.

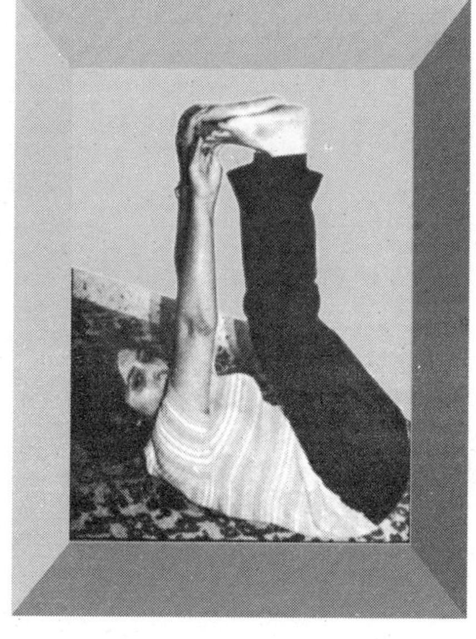

4. Lie down on the ground, lift both legs. Lift your head and try to hold toes so that the entire burden is centred on the waist.

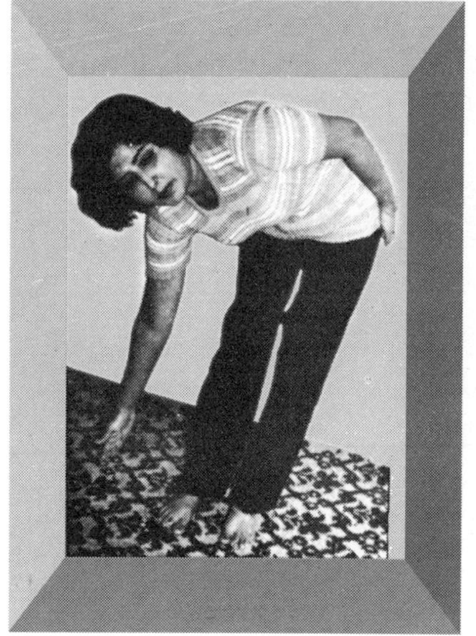

5. Stand straight. Bend to the right slowly and touch ground. Come up and straighten yourself. Now bend towards left.

***

30. SHAPELY HIPS AND THIGHS

You may have a beautiful face, but if your body is disproportionate, your personality will lose all its appeal. Usually, women have a tendency to put on fat on the hips. Fat hips and flabby thighs spoil the gait. One becomes lethargic and the body looks ugly. Obesity gives rise to various ailments and ailments prevent one from exercising. It is, therefore, important to be alert. Obesity does not occur suddenly. It is a gradual process and hence a beauty-conscious woman recognises the signals at the very beginning and takes steps to keep her body in shape. If she takes early measures, she will not find it difficult to maintain her body. Every woman must know the required proportions of her thighs and hips according to her height :

Correct Proportion of Hips and Thighs (in cm)		
Height	Hips	Thighs
153	86	47
155.5	86	48.5
158	87.5	51
160.5	89	52
163	91.5	53
165.5	94	54.5
168	95	56

This table shows the correct, balanced measurement. If you find you do not fit into it, take care. A little precaution, a few exercises and dieting will help you reduce.

Precautions

Our food habits in general are responsible for our obesity. We eat fried food, *ghee* with *dal* and *chapatti*. We do not exercise regularly. Consequently, we put on weight. The first signal of weight gain comes when the hips become fat. The first step is to avoid greasy and fried food. Do not drink water in the middle of your meal, either drink it before or after a meal. Take a walk after dinner. Going to bed or sitting immediately after meals is one of the causes of flabbiness, particularly of hips and stomach. Take a light mid-day meal. Dieting is an effective measure to reduce, but dieting does not mean skipping meals or going hungry. These extreme steps are harmful. They leave the body weak and deform the figure. Obesity cannot be reduced overnight. So, one must be patient and take gradual measures.

Massages

Hips and thighs can be given proper shape with massages. In Western countries massage parlours are abundant and our country is also not far behind. Most five-star hotels have 'health clubs' with massage facility. However the best is to use home methods. Massage activates the thighs and hips, relaxes the body and removes tension. The best time for massaging is in the morning after toilet and before bath. But, if this does not suit your routine, you can do it at night before going to bed. Mustard oil, olive oil or massage cream can be used.

Electric massagers are also available in the market which are effective, but the best is to massage with hands. The various methods used for massaging with hands are stroking, kneading, pinching, squeezing, patting, rolling. It would be done slowly and then rapidly. Massage should start with the knees and move upwards to the hips. 'Iodized jelly' is beneficial for hip massage. Hips must be kneaded first and then stroked. Stroking should be in half-circular motion and move fast towards waist. Massage daily for 10 minutes.

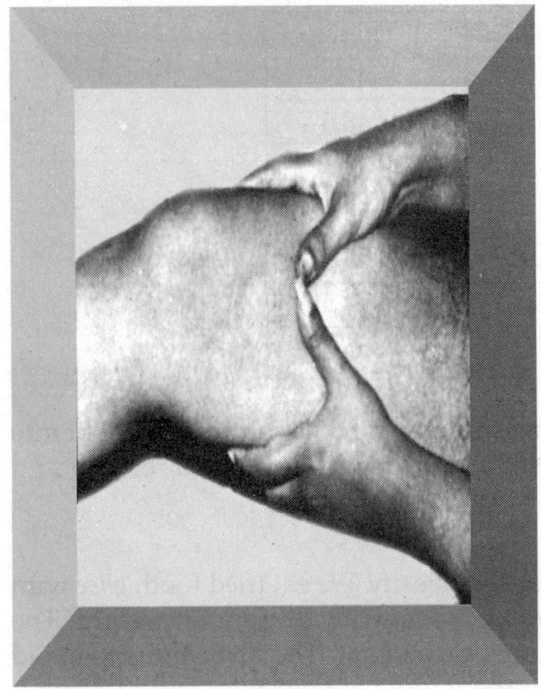

Storking

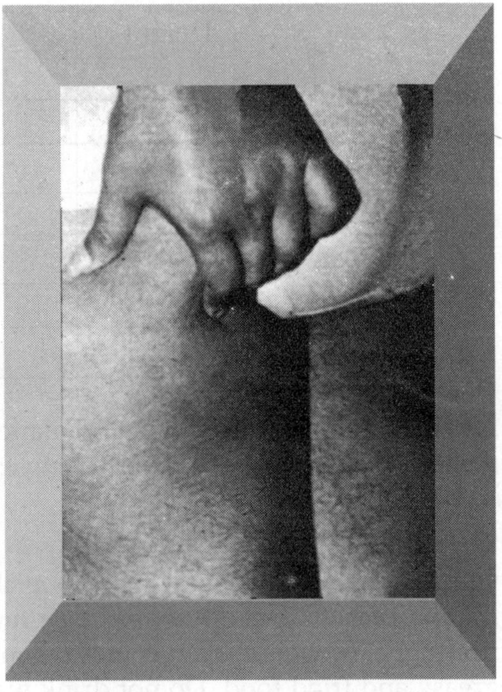

Kneeding

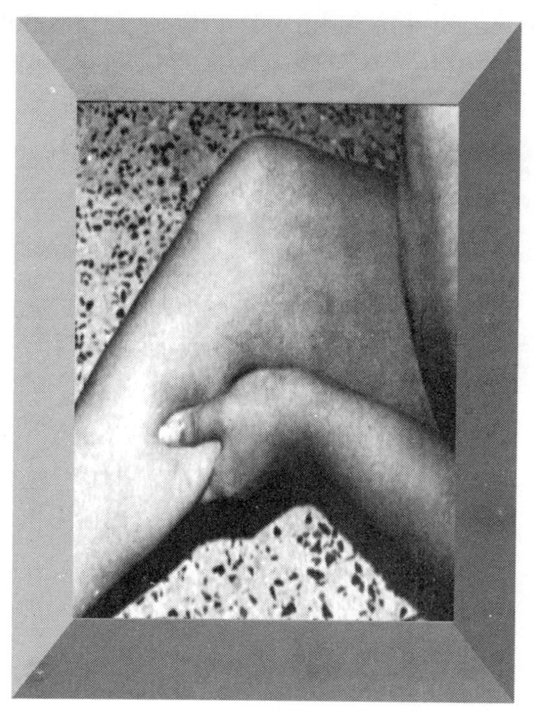

Rolling

Patting

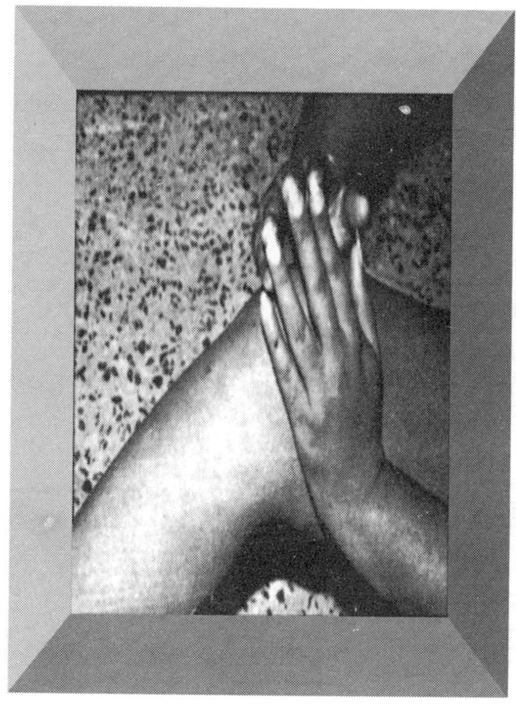

Squezing

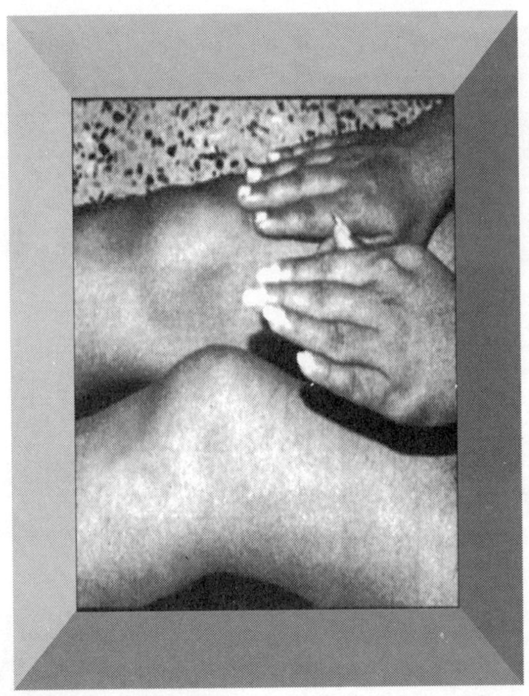

Clapping

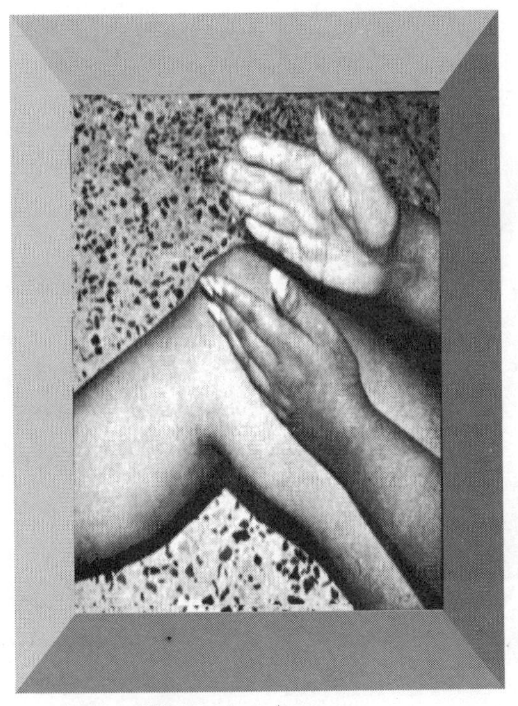

Chopping

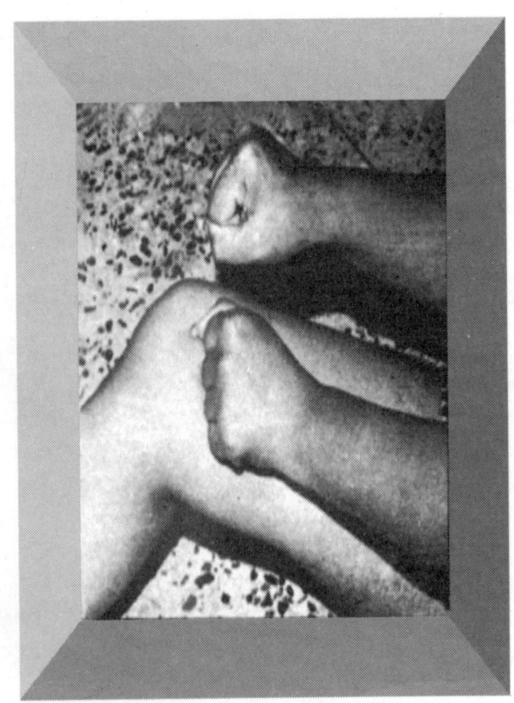

Rapping

Exercises

Exercises are essential for a shapely figure, and for an active body. A brisk walk in the fresh morning air is beneficial. Brisk walk gives exercise to bath hips and thighs. Outdoor games and swimming too are useful for toning of muscles. Exercises prevent accumulation of fat. Here are some exercises for strong and well-built thighs and hips:

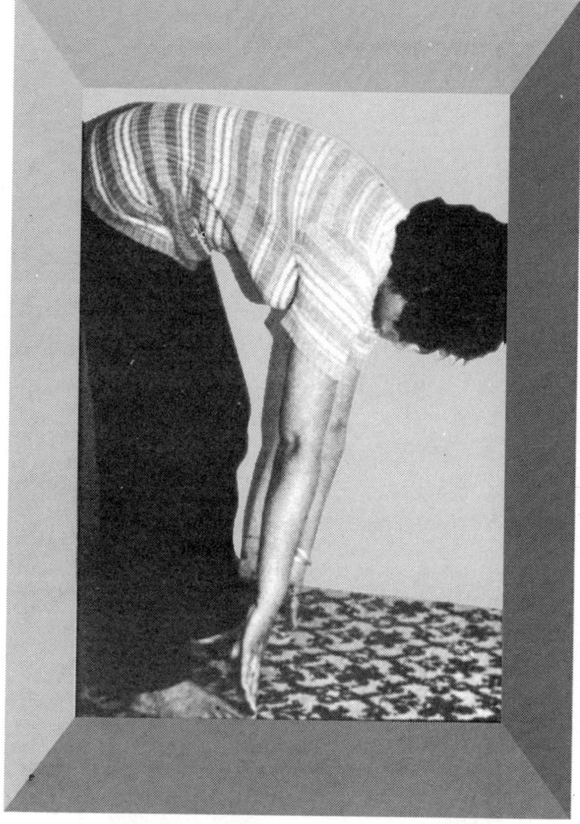

Exercise 1: Lie down on your back and make cycling movement with your legs for 10 minutes.

Exercise 2: Lie down on your back and stretch both arms parallel on the ground. Lift up right knee and bend it towards your chest. Take it to normal position. Repeat it with left leg. Do it for 5-10 minutes.

Exercise 3: Stand straight and stretch the feet about half a metre. Bend forward slowly to touch toes. Stay in this position for twenty seconds. Come back to normal position. Repeat 10 times.

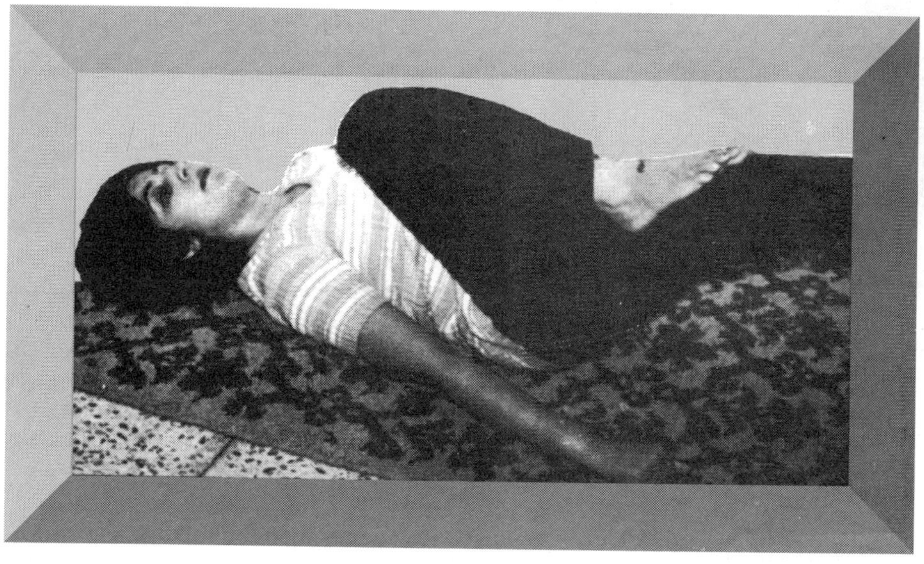

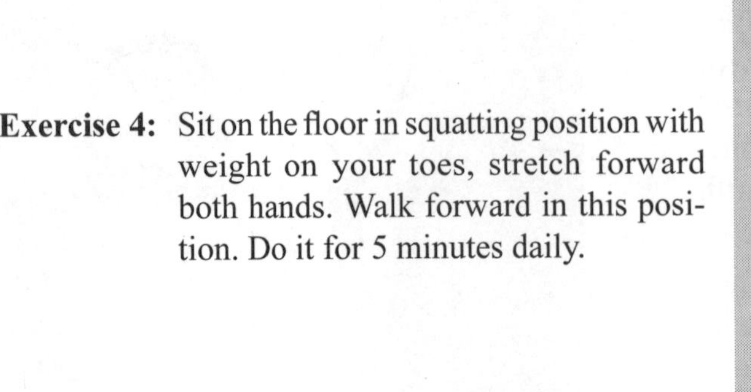

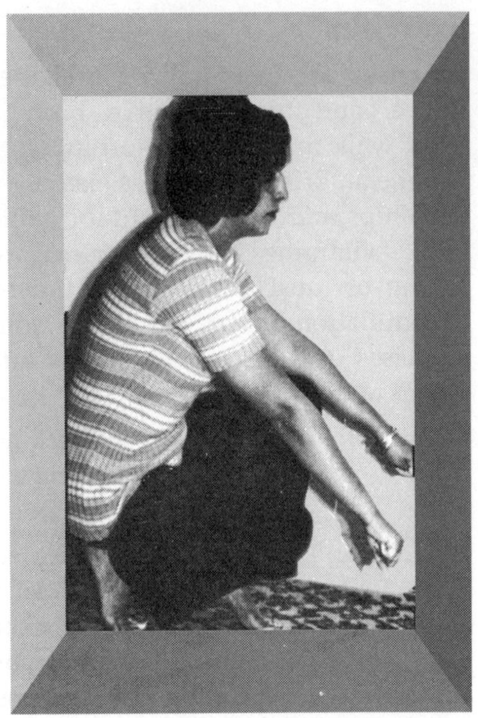

Exercise 4: Sit on the floor in squatting position with weight on your toes, stretch forward both hands. Walk forward in this position. Do it for 5 minutes daily.

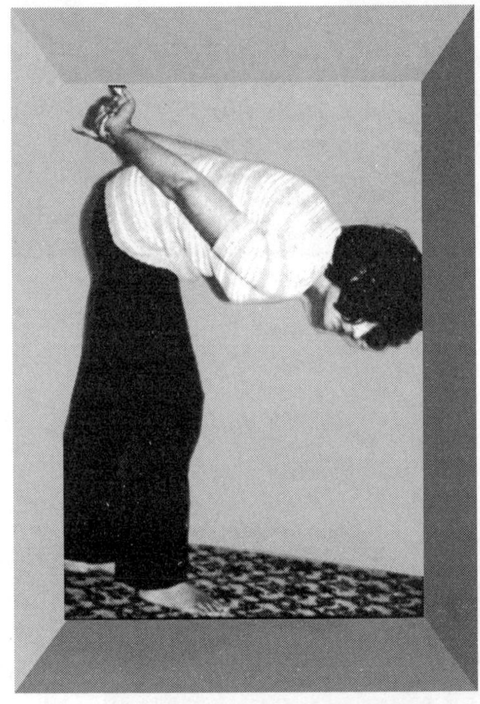

***Exercise 5*:** Stand straight joining your heels. Take a step forward and bend with it as much as you can. Keep your arms tucked at your back. Bring the forward step back and stand in original position. Repeat it with left leg. It is good for calves.

Note: To begin with, do these exercises 2-3 times each and not for longer duration. Increase slowly. Exercises should be done in open air. It will give clean air and oxygen to the body.

31. SHAPELY ARMS

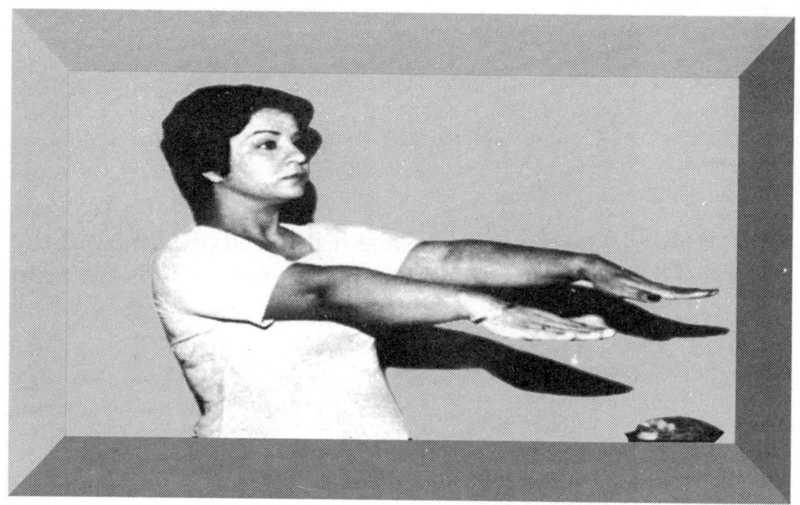

The fashion of sleeveless blouses, shirts, maxis and kaftan requires extra-attention to be paid to the arms which stay exposed in these attires. Slackness in maintaining shapely arms result in loosing the charm of your outfit. All your efforts to look smart and modern goes waste. Some sore points are: very fat arms, hairy forearms, very thin and flabby arms. Likewise, shapelessness, dryness and scragginess mar the beauty. Sleeveless dresses expose their ugliness, giving an unattractive impression of the entire personality. Here are a few suggestions for ensuring their beauty:

Arms are important for your body and a couple of minutes a day spent caring for them can be worthwhile. You must ensure if you have arms which are naturally balanced in shape. If they are flabby and have unwanted fat and flesh, try swimming, grinding with hands (*chakki*), badminton. Or choose some light weight exercise which will give maximum movement to the arms. If your arms are thin, you can increase intake of fat contents and protein in food. Massage with til (linseed) oil is also useful.

Unwanted hair on the forearms should not be neglected. They should be removed. There are many methods for removing hair which can be used. If arms are dry, rub in salt on them. Before bath, moisten the arms, take a fistful of salt and rub it in circular motion. Another method is to make a paste with oat flour and milk. Massage the paste on the dry part, leave for 15 minutes and wash off. Skin becomes soft and clean.

Yet another method for beautiful arms is as follows:

Take 1 spoonful of tomato juice, 1 spoonful lemon juice and 1 spoonful milk. Mix these well and rub on arms. Leave for 15 minutes. Wash off. In winter the oil secreting glands become inactive which results in dryness of the skin. Take a little milk, add olive oil and a few drops of rose water and massage on the arms. Take bath after 15 minutes.

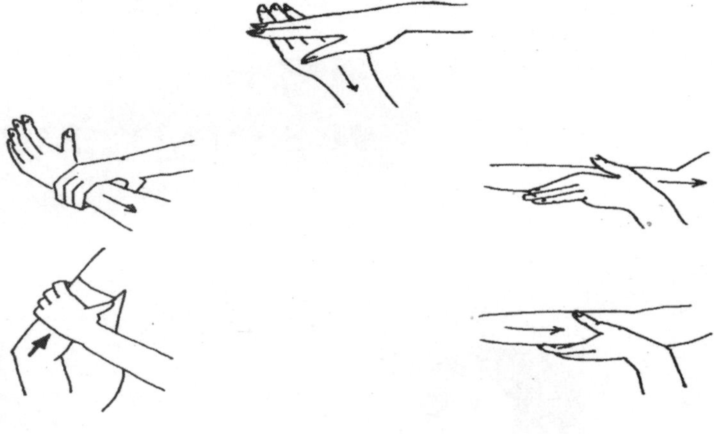

Elbows are also most often neglected. They become dry, hard and black. Avoid placing elbows on chair or table as far as possible. Scrub them well while bathing. You can use a stone scrubber to clean them. A simple method to clean elbows and make them soft is to take a lemon, slice it into halves, take out the juice, place them on the table and sit placing your elbows within these shells. You can sit in this pose for 10-15 minutes

***

32. BEAUTIFUL FINGERS

Hands are the symbols of beauty as well as messengers of sentiments. Possibly, they are more important than the beauty of the face. A beautiful face gives pleasure to the eyes but beautiful hands give the pleasure of touch and sight. There are 3 things that keep hands beautiful: Soft skin, shapely fingers and beautiful nails. Household chores done with hands, make them rough, spoil the shape of fingers and crack nails. These chores are cleaning utensils, laundering, gardening, cleaning and chopping vegetables and brooming and mopping.

Care for your Hands

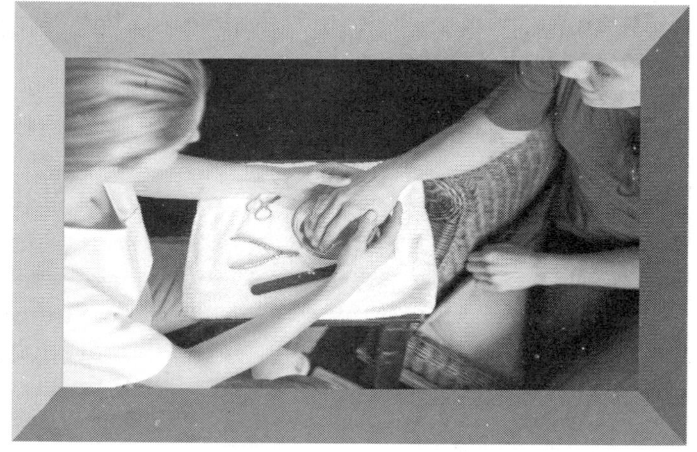

Cleaning utensils requires the use of detergent, lime, alongwith water. They make hands rough. Detergent powders and soaps have chemicals like caustic-soda which crack the skin and damage it by destroying the natural oils. Our skin remains greasy because of the presence of oil and sweat glands underneath. If the oil gland stops secreting oil, the skin becomes rough and abrasive. It develops redness and cracks. That, however, does not mean that women should stop household chores altogether. What is required is precaution. Wash your hands with clean water after laundering or washing utensils, apply vaseline or cold cream. Also use a mixture of rose water, glycerine and lemon juice. These help in retaining natural oils. Since our country has extreme climates— severe cold in winters, heat waves in summers and dampness in rainy season — the skin is adversely affected.

Beauty of Nails: Manicure

Manicure is essential for beautiful nails. Just as beautiful teeth are important for a beautiful face, beauty of hands has much to do with nails. Dip your fingers in soap-water for 5 minutes and clean with brush (see illustration). Add a pinch of borax or oat flour to give extra softness.

Use cuticle pusher to push back dead skin.

Give shape to the nails by rubbing with emery board. Give crescent shape with nail filer. Nail filing should be done in one direction. Rubbing in the opposite direction makes the end rough and uneven. If nails become hot while filing, dip them in tepid oil to keep them soft. Do not dip fingers in oil before nail filing because nails get brittle and they break. After filing, wash with lukewarm water and dry.

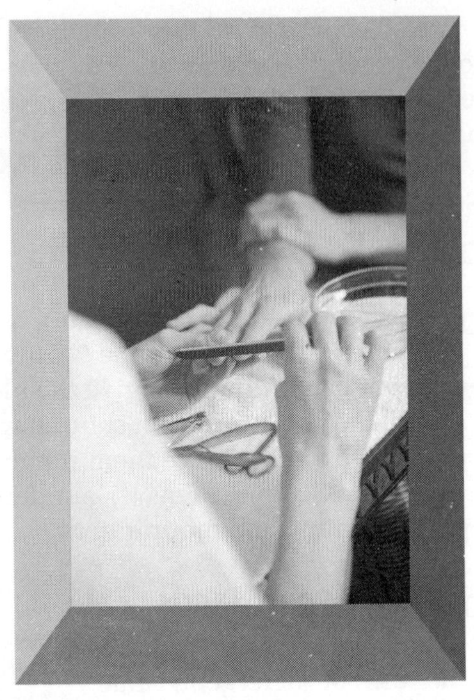

Massage nails with cold cream at night. Nails break at night when they entangle in sheets, etc. It is, therefore, necessary to preserve them. For longer nails plastic caps are available. A special varnish is available for the protection of nails. Nail polish is also a good preserver. Rubbing lemon peel is also effective for ensuring strong nails. To keep them soft and flexible, cuticle cream can be used at night before going to bed. All the implements used in manicure are shown in the following illustration.

Applying Nail Polish

Rest your arm on a table so that the hands do not shake while applying nail polish. Remove all grease from nails. Shake well the nail polish bottle and apply with brush from the root of nails to their tips. Leave it for 5 minutes to dry. Apply a second coat. It gives shine. Polish should not spread to the skin around the nails. Nail polish tends to get air bubbles when the bottle is shaken often, and it also clots. This spoils the polish. It then cannot be applied evenly.

For polishing, first apply it on the sides and fill in the middle carefully. This will prevent it from spreading to the sides. In order to bring extra shine on the nails varnish can be applied for 12 hours before using nail polish. In rainy season, it takes longer to dry. Remember to remove nail polish once a week for nails to breathe. Use only standard products. Sub-standard nail polishes may harm the roots of nails.

Nails can be given the desired shape with nail polish. For example, if you want them to look roundish, do not use nail polish on sides. They can be made to look oblong, by leaving out the elevated corners without nail polish. If both edges are left without polish, nails look smaller in size.

Some Tips for Beautiful Hands

- Take milk cream, add a few drops of lemon juice and glycerine. Rub on hands at night.
- Wash hands with vinegar mixed water or lemon juice mixed water to ward off the ill-effects of hot water, soda, soap, and other detergents.
- Glycerine, mixed with rose water or cucumber juice should be rubbed on hands with a cotton wool swab. It cleans the skin.
- Massage hands and fingers with almond oil at night before going to bed. It makes skin attractive.
- Use hand lotion in winter to avoid winter-dryness. If your skin is too dry, add carbolic acid to vaseline and rub in.
- If hands are rough, take a spoonful of sugar and lemon juice. Rub palms till sugar dissolves. Wash off with cold water. Honey can be used instead of sugar. Boil potatoes. Peel them before they get cold. Pulp them well and rub the pulp on fingers.
- Hairy hands look ugly. These hair can be removed by waxing, or hidden by bleaching. Bleach or wax once a month.

***

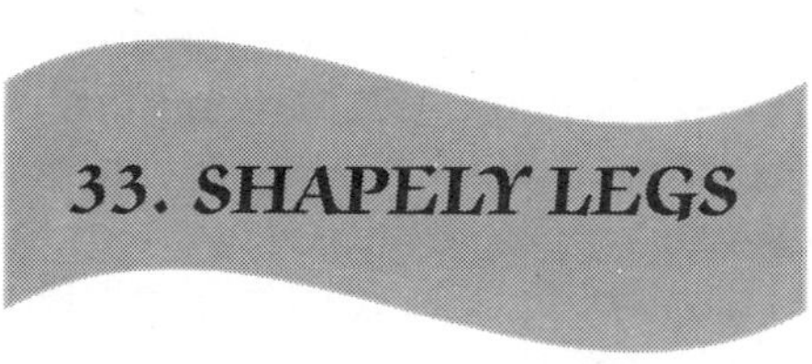

33. SHAPELY LEGS

A perfect beauty is flawless from top to toe. Usually, in our concept of beauty we pay more attention to the face, hair, hands, dress, and jewellery. Feet are often neglected. That is the reason why many times a well-dressed woman tries to hide her feet. A little care of feet and legs alongwith simple exercises can save you from an embarrassing situation.

Healthy Feet

Rough feet can be tended by dipping them in hot water mixed with a little soda-bicarbonate. Scrub the rough parts and heels with pumice-stone. Tender parts like toes should be scrubbed with a nylon brush. Wipe your feet with a clean, dry towel and sprinkle a good amount talcum powder on them.

Nails should be cut straight and oil must be applied on their tips. Rub with a filer and make them even. Do not cut nails too deep otherwise they will appear too short and the nail polish will look ugly on them. Now, wash again, wipe and massage them with cold cream.

Feet have a tendency to sweat profusely. If you wear shoes and socks, then they stink. Sweat dries the skin. Dry parts should be rubbed well with cold cream. Sprinkle some deodorant between the toes. Do not wear the same sandals or shoes throughout the day. You can change shoes, sandals, if possible. This is refreshing. Wear clean socks and wash them after each wear.

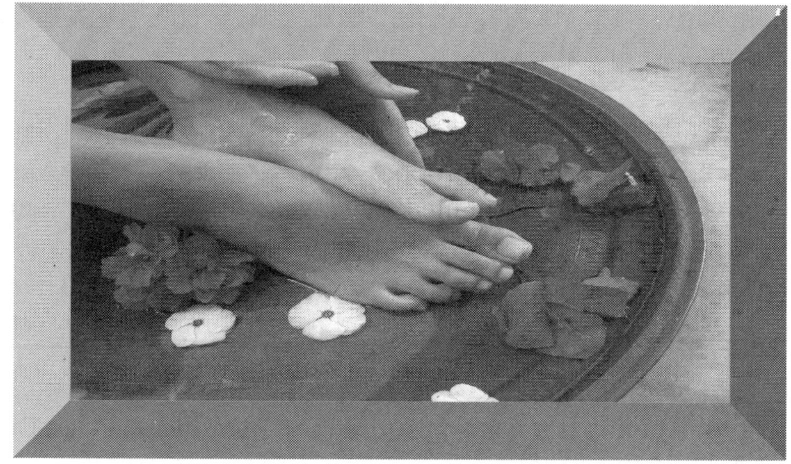

Healthy Feet

Women often complain of swelling on their feet, tiredness and itching. For swelling, an effective remedy is to massage them with lemon juice or camphor spirit and give them rest for 15 minutes. If itching, wash frequently, dry them and sprinkle talcum powder. If feet remain tired and worn (fatigued), walk on the toes, pour hot water on the feet for 1 minute followed by cold water for 1 minute. Dry well and massage gently from the heels upward to the knees. It is an effective remedy to remove weariness.

Some women have problem with cracked heels. This is common with those who wear sandals and open chapals. Cracked heels are not only painful but also ugly to look at. Soak a piece of bread in a little milk, add a few drops of almond oil and rub on the cracked part.

Knots (corns) on Feet

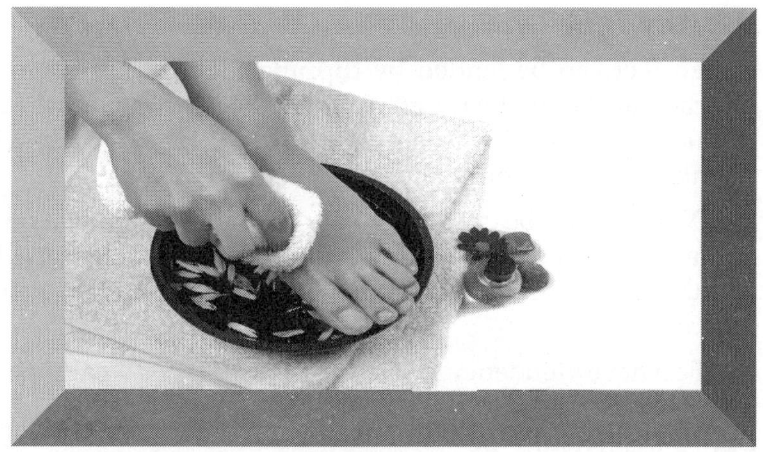

Correct choice of shoes or footwear is essential, for tight shoes or sandals leave knotty corns on the soles of the feet, toes and heels. While buying your shoes see to it that the design is comfortable and the leather is soft. Corns are painful and affect the gait. Moreover, walking barefoot during domestic chores leave the soles of feet dry and hard, giving rise to corns.

To avert corns, keep the feet clean. Corns become septic if not looked after well. Consult a beautician or chiropodist in case of corns. If these are not too old or hard it is easy to treat them. Use of medicated 'corn caps' is effective in removing them.

Hard corns can be treated thus: Take lukewarm water in a basin, add some shampoo and make lather with shampoo. Add salt, soda-bicarb and hydrogen peroxide to it and soak feet in this mixture for half an hour. Corns become soft. Take out your feet and wipe well. Massage corns tightly to soften them more. Now, scratch with a 'scrabbler'. A scrabbler is a kind of steel knife. It should be treated with an anti-septic before use. After scrabbling use some anti-septic lotion or disinfectant. Do not remove a corn with a scrabbler in one stroke, it may leave a wound. This process can be repeated after a day or two. Thus, corns become loose and can be removed easily.

Some home remedies are as follows:

- Apply glycerine on heels and toes and wash off after half an hour.

➤ Rub honey before taking bath and wash off after half an hour.
➤ Regular exercise strengthen the feet muscles and regulate blood circulation.

Maintenance of Toe Nails

Maintenance of feet and their cleanliness is known as 'pedicure'. Pedicure can be done at home or at a beauty parlour. Take lukewarm water in a basin, add a little shampoo, a pinch of soda-bicarb and a few drops of hydrogen peroxide to it. Remove nail polish with a nail polish remover. Dip your feet in this water. Rub nails and clean them. Clean heels with a pumice-stone. Wipe dry. Give shape to the nails and rub with a filer to a round shape. Clean nails, their tips and sides with cotton wool wrapped on orange-stick. Rub oil on the nails so that it soaks in. It keeps the nail healthy and the cuticle soft. Push back the dead skin with a pusher or the flat end of the orange-stick. Then rub it with sand-paper or cut it with scissors.

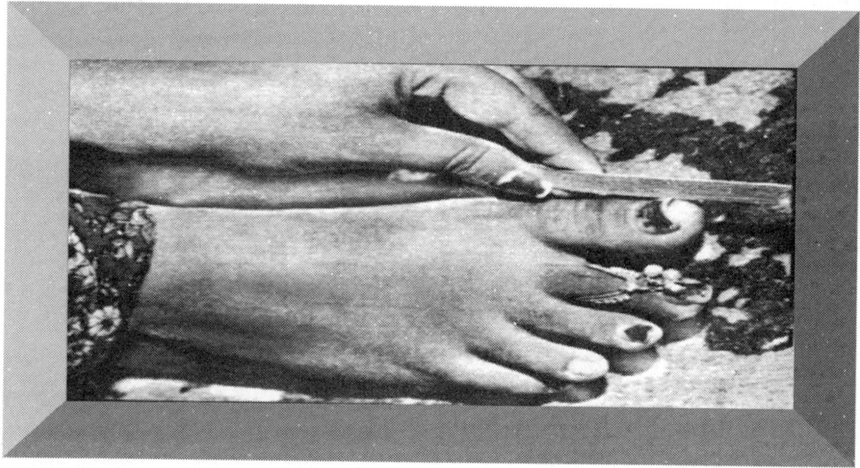

Wipe off the grease before applying nail polish. You can use nail polish remover.

Apply nail polish once, let it dry and apply a second coat. You can place small cotton wool pads between your toes to facilitate quick movement of the nail polish brush. Moreover, nail polish does not stick to the skin around. Nail polish is available in many shades but choose the one which goes with your complexion.

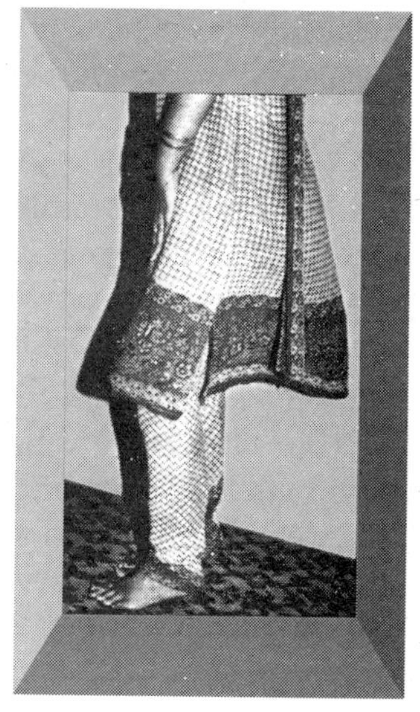

Simple Exercises for Feet

Exercise 1: Stand straight. Join the heels and lift up the big toe at 45° angle. Keep knees straight, take your arms up and keep straight. Stand on your toes lifting heels for some time and bend forward bringing your arms in front.

Do not let your heels touch the ground while bending. Repeat 5 times. Inhale while coming up and exhale while going down. If it is uncomfortable to lift arms you can place them on the hips. This exercise strengthens the muscles of the forepart of the feet, heels and legs.

Exercise 2: Sit at a high place, lift the legs keeping knees straight. Now move each feet in a circular motion first clockwise, then anti-clockwise. Repeat several times.

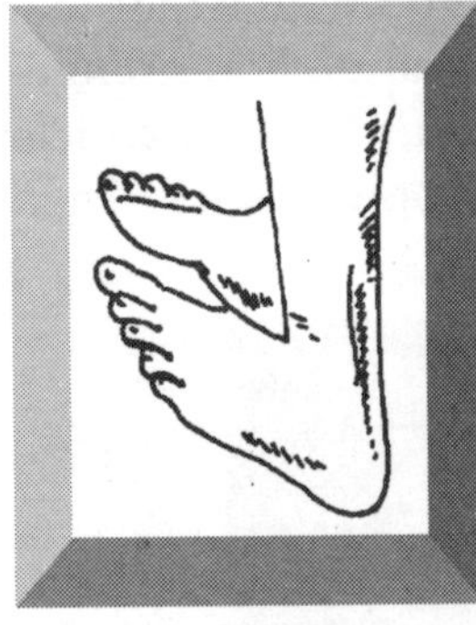

Exercise 3: Sit at a high place and lift your legs. Keep knees straight. Bend feet from ankles toward leg-side. Come to original position. Repeat 10 to 15 times. It is good for forefeet, toes and legs.

Massage for Legs

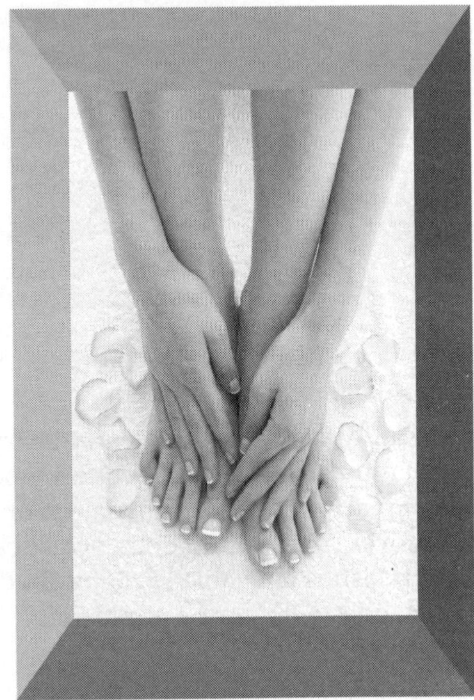

Massage is an effective method to increase the beauty of legs. Massaging is simple and beneficial. It burns the extra fat, strengthens muscles and increases the capacity of various organs. Spare some time for massage after your morning exercises. Massage the legs 3-4 minutes. It should be done slowly and steadily but firmly, because if rubbed too hard, the skin peels off and gets marked. Do not be in a hurry while massaging. Take oil on your finger tips and massage, using different methods like patting, stroking, bending. End it with patting. Take bath after a massage, wipe with a thick towel and sprinkle powder. In the beginning, it is hard to massage fast but with practice hands move speedily and flexibly.

Caress slowly the massaged portion. It softens the skin and relieves taut nerves. Massage should begin slowly followed by rapid movements. The position of hands should be relaxed. Massage should start from the ankles, through calves and move towards knees. Various methods such stroking, kneading, squeezing, patting, clapping, wrapping should be followed.

Pressing the Body

Massage by pressing does not mean that you should hurt yourself. It is done to stimulate blood circulation in legs. Muscles and tissues can be held in pinch and pressed. The motion should be from down to up.

Pressing during massage removes swelling. Press the part with both palms as if massaging with both hands.

Press the sides of the legs and the calves. Move hands towards the hips. Use cream as a lubricant. Apply circular motions with the palms on the hips. Massaging shows its effect quite soon.

34. BATHING – KEEP IT FRESH

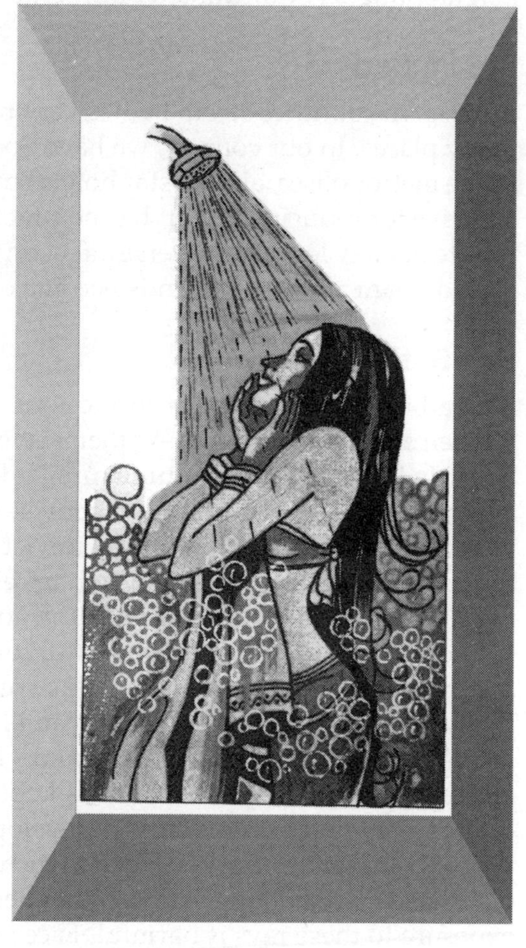

You are a lucky one if you have clean, beautiful, soft and lustrous skin. But, is there any guarantee that it will last forever? What is bequeathed to you by nature is your treasure and you have to preserve it, for which you have to make efforts.

Bath is an effective beauty therapy. It is important not only for cleanliness but also for the skin. If you are using soap, do not use very hot water. It will damage the oil glands. Fresh, lukewarm water is best for taking bath. Apply soap on the exposed parts to remove dirt and dust particles. Use water in plenty, do not be economical in your use of water. Towel should be clean, soft and puffy. Ascertain before wiping that you have washed off all soap. Wipe with towel by dabbing and then rubbing gently. Do not rub the towel on tender parts such as face, neck, chin and stomach otherwise wrinkles will appear.

In case of any skin disease use a medicated, disinfectant soap available with chemists. Ordinary soaps are not disinfectant. In summer, take bathe twice a day to wash off the sweat and grease. Some vital natural oils are destroyed in the process of taking bath, but the body recoups them soon. Use of soaps should be discontinued in case of dry skin, in winter and in advanced age. If at all soap is to be used, choose a glycerine soap. Perfumed soap or caustic-soda soap should be avoided. Remember that soap is for cleanliness and not for beauty. Start soaping the body from head, come down to face, neck, shoulders, underarms, arms, waist, thighs, legs and face.

Bath can be taken in running water, standing water, in tubs, under shower or with steam. Bathing in the running river water is very beneficial. Tub-bath is more a fashion than beneficial. When we sit in a tub all our body dirt dissolves in the water but sticks onto our body again. The very purpose of taking bath is defeated in case of tub-bath. Bathing under tap-water or shower is good for removing dirt.

Sandalwood paste keeps the body mildly fragrant and refreshed throughout the day. For this, take sandalwood paste, mix rosewater. Make a paste and apply a thick coat. Leave it on for 15 minutes, let it dry and then take a bath. To lighten a dark complexion, a simple home remedy is: take oat flour tied in a kerchief or napkin, dip it in unboiled (raw) milk and rub on the body twice a week. Slowly the skin acquires a lighter tinge. For unwanted hair, scrub with gram flour (besan).

Steam Bath

In Western countries steam bath is very popular. There are public steam-bathrooms at many places. In our country, we have Spas which are now found every health where. In the metropolises, all five-star hotels have health clubs with steam bath facilities. It is effective for reducing fat but has no practical utility as it does not clean the skin. Very hot steam may leave an adverse effect on the heart. Blood vessels expand permanently due to steam and sweat glands become overactive.

Sun Bath

Sunbathing is very popular in Western countries. It is a common sight to find men, women and children exposing themselves to the sun on beaches, in hotels or in health clubs. In India, because of our naturally dark complexion, sun bathing is often avoided and rather it causes tanning. Moreover, since our climate is not cold all through the year, sun-bath is not a necessity. A Soviet scientist Nicholas Salus has established after research that sun-rays affect the white cells the most. Boston Medical Research Centre has attested the finding. For a healthy and clear skin, sun-rays play a significant role. Without exposure to sun the harmful foreign matter will accumulate under the skin. Sun-rays are essential for animal as well as plant life. No plant can grow without the warmth of the sun, no flower can bloom, nor any fruit can ripe without it. Rays of the sun are a rich source of vitamin D which strengthens the body with calcium and phosphorus. When a man was kept away from the rays of the Sun for a couple of months, as an experiment, he developed skin abrasion and boils. Sun-rays give a protective shield to the body which increases resistance to diseases. For pimples and blackheads, sunbathing is recommended. It is good for all skin diseases. But, long exposure to these rays is harmful. Face and head should be covered while other parts of the body could be exposed. Too much exposure can activate the brain adversely. It can cause wrinkles and falling of hair. It is advisable to drink one litre water with a lemon or two squeezed in it (*nimbu-pani*).

35. EATING A BALANCED DIET

Obesity is an enemy of beauty. It destroys the shapeliness of the body and gives it an unpleasant look. People think of it to be a disease. However, obesity is not an illness in itself, but is a foster-mother of various diseases. A shapely figure can be maintained with the help of a regular balanced diet and daily exercises. Heaviness of the body hinders the free and healthy flow of blood through the veins and muscles. This in turn affects the functioning of the heart, leading to heart problems, blood pressure, diabetes and other diseases. A 10 per cent extra fat means a risk of reduced longevity by 20 per cent.

What is Dieting?

Dieting signifies the intake of a balanced diet; and a balanced diet means the kind of food which guarantees good health. Nourishing diet contains protein, carbohydrates fats and vitamins & minerals. Dieting does not mean starving. It means controlling the weight through a balanced diet. It is necessary to consult a doctor before going on a a in order to ascertain that we do not take drastic measures in lose weight. It is also advisable to avoid the in long run take of weight-reducing drugs. These drugs may prove effective initially but in the congrua they prove to be harmful.

Your Diet

Normally a healthy body digests food within 15-20 minutes and converts it into energy. A wise and correct choice of food items, the method of cooking them and punctuality and regularity of food timings are important for good health. A sound health in itself is a means to real beauty. Our diet must contain a balanced proportion of protein and carbohydrates. A young woman of an average height, who is not pregnant, or who is not engaged in physical labour, requires 2300 calories a day. One gram protein gives 4 calories, 1 gram carbohydrate also gives 4 calories, whereas 1 gram of fat gives 9 calories.

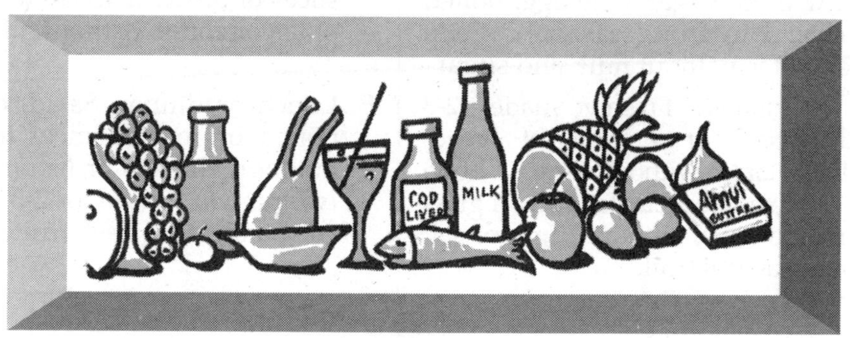

Protein

It is found in abundance in milk, eggs, meat and fish, soyabean, almond, coconut, groundnut, etc. It gives us strength.

Carbohydrates

It is found in cereals, vegetables, fruits, etc. It helps in generating calories. Deficiency of carbohydrates leads to weakness.

Fat

One of the 3 nutrients (along with carbohydrates and proteins) that supply calories & the body. It provides calcium to the tissues and is important for growth.

Suggestions

- For raw (uncooked) salad, use tomato, carrot, beet-root, radish, cucumber, *kakdi*, green-leaby vegetables such as *palak*, soya, etc., and onion.
- Grapes, pomegranadtes, mussambi, apples, pear, apricot, strawberry, papaya, water-melon and pineapple are nourishing and good for checking obesity.
- Instead of sugar, use pure honey or khand sari.
- Use as little water as you can for cooking vegetables. Steaming is better. Overcooking for longer duration causes loss of some vital vitamins. Intake of sufficient quantity of fresh water is advisable because it helps in regulating bowel movement which gives an attractive glow to skin.

DIET CHART	
Vegetarian Diet Ratio of calories : Protein — 30% Carbohydrates — 65% Fat — 5%	Non-vegetarian Diet Ratio of calories: Protein — 30% Carbohydrates — 50% Fats — 20%
A. Breakfast: Slices of 250 grams bread with butter, jam or jelly. Oat meal cornflakes in milk without sugar. One egg, boiled or poached. Any fruit (seasonal). A cup of tea or coffee without milk and sugar. B. Lunch or dinner: Freshly made, 2-3 roasted *chapatis* or 4 slices of bread, cooked vegetables without spices, 1 bowl (*katori*) of curried vegetable, 1 small glass butter-milk or curd without sugar or salt and some seasonal fruit.	A. Breakfast: Some fruit or a cup of fresh fruit-juice, 1 egg (poached or boiled), 2 slices of bread with jam or butter, a cup of tea or coffee without milk and sugar. B. Lunch or dinner: Salad, chicken soup, boiled or roasted meat (one piece) or tandoori chicken or fish (not more than two pieces), 1 *naan*, or 2-3 *chapatis*, plain curd and some fresh fruit (seasonal).

***

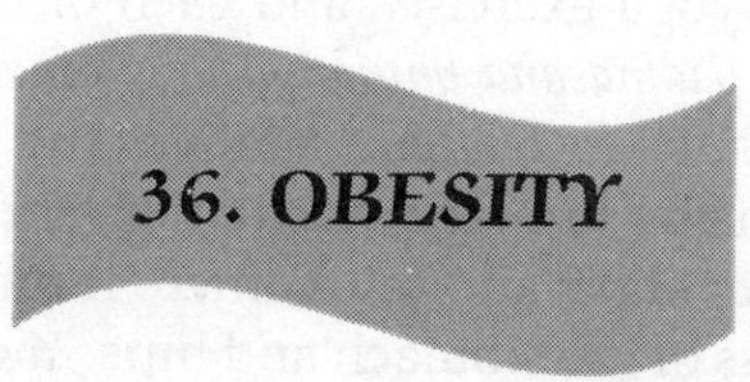

36. OBESITY

Obesity is not a disease in itself but it is the root of many diseases such as high blood pressure, heart trouble, diabetes, kidney problems, gout and joint-pain, kidney and gall bladder stone, skin diseases. Regular exercise and massage are effective in controlling fatness; likewise, balanced diet, yoga practice and other mechanical devices are also very beneficial. We have already discussed various exercises and ways of massages in the previous chapters. Here, we shall focus on obesity, its causes, kinds and the methods to control it.

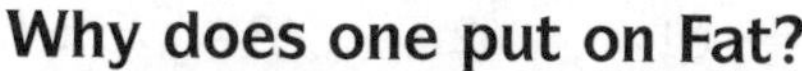

Why does one put on Fat?

- Of the many causes of obesity, the main is overeating, lack of exercise and lethargy. Another cause can be traced back to heredity. Usually, fat parents have fat children.
- Overactive glands increase appetite and multiply the fat contents in the body.
- Imbalance of hormones in the body also results in obesity. The body develops the tendency to put on fat. A constant rise in weight is the result of the decrease of thyroid hormones and increase of insulin hormone.
- Mental tension, frustration, loneliness and other phobia also cause obesity.
- Women put on weight after child-birth if they do not exercise.

Types of Obesity

Obesity can be divided roughly into 3 categories — i) fatty overweight, ii) watery overweight and iii) cellulitis.

Fatty overweight causes flabbiness all over the body. Watery overweight occurs in women in which the lower part of the body becomes fat. Cellulitis is the result of chemical reaction. It affects only some parts of body like forehead, lower part of face, back of the neck, chin, elbows, legs, knees and hips. Cellulitis also causes pain and swelling of joints.

Yoga is an effective means to keep the body weight balanced and enhance facial glow. There are 84 types of yoga exercises and each of these has its importance and effect. But, some of them like *padmasana, bhujangasana, konasana, ushtrasana* and *yogasana* are effective for physical beauty. *Padmasana* removes the deficiencies and deformities of the spine. *Bhujangasana* helps in blood circulation and increases beauty. *Konasana* is specially recommended for short and fat women. It maintains balance of the body. *Ushtrasana* reduces flabbiness of the stomach and hips. *Yogasana* is beneficial for young and middle-aged women. It gives psychological pep and increases mental beauty.

Mechanical gadget for reducing weight are gaining popularity these days. They are also effective in controlling and reducing obesity. These can be bought and used at home.

Weight-chart according to Height and Age

Age	15-19	20-24	25-29	30-34	35-39	40-44	45-49	50-59	60 +
Height (in cm)	Weight (in Kilograms)								
152.5	49	51	52	54	55	57	58	59	59
155	51	52	54	55	56	58	59	60	61
157.5	52	53	55	56	58	59	61	62	63
160	54	54	57	57	59	61	62	63	64
162.5	55	56	57	59	61	62	64	65	66
165	56	57	59	60	63	64	65	66	67
167.5	57	59	60	63	64	66	67	68	69

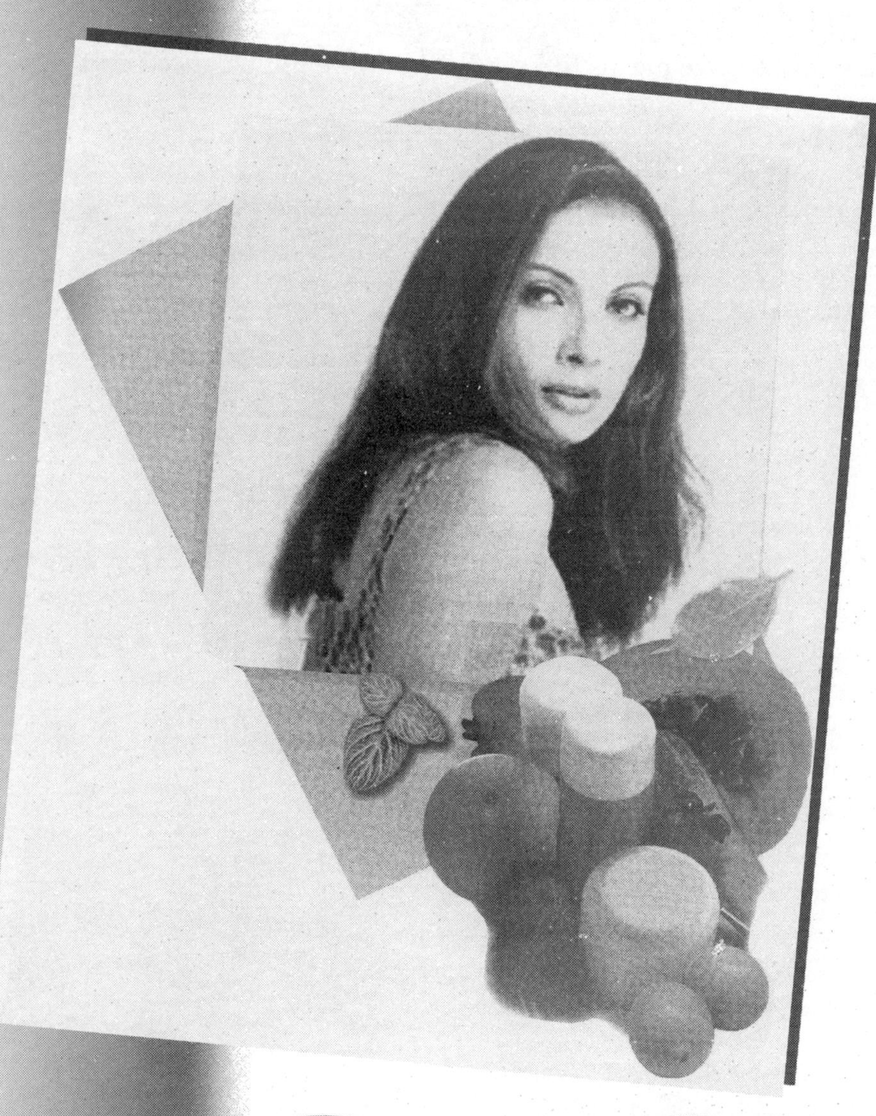

PART 5
HOME-MADE BEAUTY PRODUCTS

37. EAT WELL TO LOOK BEAUTIFUL

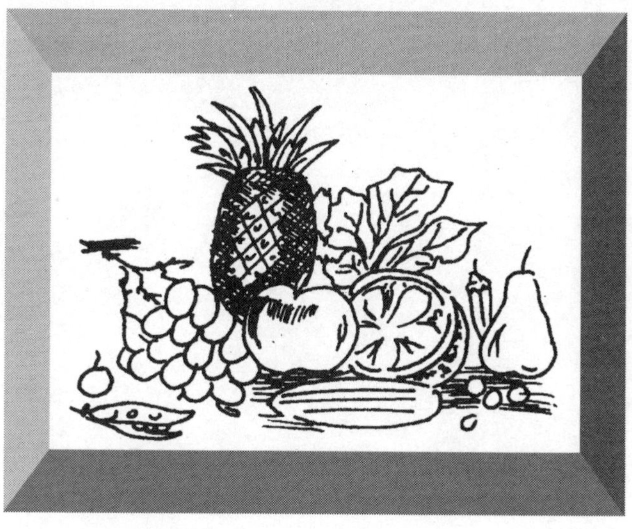

In ancient times, women became conscious of their beauty as soon as they entered adolescence; beauty-aids and cosmetics were not as easily available to them as they are today. So, they cared for their looks with natural products–fruits and vegetables. It was not only an effective means to maintain their beauty, but was also inexpensive. Natural things are, indeed, the best bet for beauty. Banana, apple, orange, water-melon, raspberry, etc., are effective beauty-aids. If you have dry skin, take a banana, mash it, add a spoonful of rose water and two drops glycerine. Store this mixture in a bottle in the fridge. Apply this before make-up, keep it for half an hour and wash it off with lukewarm water. The pulp of one banana can last a week.

It you have an oily skin, take an apple, peel it, chop it in small pieces, apply on the face like a paste coating, leave for half an hour, wash with lukewarm water. Apple is nourishing for the skin.

Are you worried because you have an unattractive skin? Then try this: Peel an orange, boil the pulpy part in clean water for 15 minutes and strain it when it gets cold. Use it as a lotion and your skin will be velvet-soft. If the skin is carped due to heat-wave, rub water melon pieces on the affected portion. Water-melon absorbs heat from your body. Raspberry juice is an effective cleansing lotion. For removing make-up, rub peeled raspberries. The juice will remove make-up and dust particles. Apply a good cold cream and massage. The skin will attain a natural glow.

Among vegetables, effective beauty-aids are lemon, potato, carrot, cucumber, tomato, et. al. For oily skin, lemon is effective. Add a small quantity of milk and lemon juice in oat flour. Apply this mixture on the face, leave it for 20 minutes and wash off with lukewarm water. This lotion removes unwanted facial hair. Lemon juice is an effective hair conditioner. If you have oily hair, rinse with water mixed with lemon juice after shampooing. For black spots and shadows, lemon juice mixed with fresh milk cream can be applied before retiring to bed. Potato also keeps the skin clean and fresh. Carrot has effective ingredients for preserving beauty. Carrot juice can be used as a lotion. An effective lotion can be made by chopping carrot into small pieces, boil them in water, mash and apply on the face for half an hour. For cleaning clogged pores, tomato juice and lemon juice can be mixed in equal quantities and apply. Cucumber juice is good as eye-drops in summer. Also, cucumber pieces can be placed on the eyes and rubbed on the face as a beauty-aid.

38. HOME-MADE COSMETICS

Ancient history is a witness to the fact that women have always prepared various home-made beauty aids to enhance their beauty. Now that cosmetics are manufactured in our country, women are increasingly inclined towards them. But, with the soaring prices of cosmetics, middle and lower middle-class women are finding it beyond their reach. Indeed, how many women can afford the luxury of visiting beauty clinics or buying expensive beauty aids? Consequently, they go in for cheaper products which ultimately prove injurious to health and beauty. People have now come to realise the importance of home remedies. These items have many advantages — they are less expensive, can be made easily and there is no fear of any chemical reaction. I often urge my clients to use home-made aids to keep their natural beauty intact. I am enumerating some recipes for making a few items at home, so that you not only save money but are also sure of the quality.

Tips for Preparing Cosmetics

- Correct ratio of different items for preparing various mixtures is very important. Below is given a chart of ratio :

60 drops	=	One teaspoon
3 teaspoons	=	One tablespoon
2 tablespoons	=	One eighth of a cup
4 tablespoons	=	One fourth of a cup
8 tablespoons	=	Half a cup
16 tablespoons	=	One cup

- High flame of heat diminishes the effect of various ingredients. Low heat is preferable. For liquifying oily substances put them in a small container or utensil, place the small utensil in a bigger one with hot water and keep it for a while.
- The raw material for manufacturing cosmetics at home should be purchased from a dispensing chemist shop.
- Prepare cosmetics in small quantities and keep the items cool in refrigerator.

Astringent Lotion

2 tablespoons honey
2 teaspoons ground coriander seeds
2 teaspoons nutmeg (jaiphul)
1 teaspoon cloves (tinpatia ghas)
4 teaspoons orange peels (small pieces)
8 tablespoons alcohol

4 tablespoons rose water
4 tablespoons orange flower juice
1/2 teaspoon benzoin
1/2 teaspoon storax

Process: Put all the ingredients in a large bottle and cover it with lid. Shake it. Thereafter for a week just shake the bottle twice a day in the mornings and evenings and keep it closed. After a week filter it into another bottle and keep in the fridge.

To prepare another kind of astringent lotion, take out the white of an egg and beat it. Then add 2 teaspoonfuls of cucumber juice and 1 teaspoonful of lemon juice. Shake it well. In case your skin is oily, then put 1 teaspoonful of alcohol in it. By adding a little benzoin tincture, the astringent lotion becomes more potent and removes wrinkles.

Cleansing Cream

1/2 tablespoon bees-wax
1 tablespoon emulsifying wax
4 tablespoons baby oil
2 tablespoons coconut oil
2 tablespoons water
1/4 teaspoon borax (Boric powder)
1 tablespoon raw milk and a few drops of perfume.

Process : Take bees-wax, emulsifying wax, baby oil and coconut oil in a small china bowl and melt it on medium heat. Heat water and boric powder in another bowl and mix it well. Add raw milk to it. Now remove both the bowls from the flame, mix the contents together and keep stirring till it gets cold. At the time of stirring add a few drops of perfume to it. The resultant thick paste is ready for use as a cream.

Skin Food

2 teaspoons bees-wax
2 teaspoons emulsifying wax
8 teaspoons almond oil
4 teaspoons lanolin
4 teaspoons coconut oil
6 teaspoons orange flower water
3 drops tincture benzoin

Process : Melt bees-wax, emulsifying wax, almond oil, lanolin and coconut oil on medium heat and simultaneously stir it. Now add orange flower water gradually but keep on stirring. When the mixture becomes thick, remove it from the heat and after getting it cold fill in a bottle.

Body Lotion

1/2 tablespoon lanolin
1 tablespoon petroleum jelly
4 tablespoons mineral oil
8 teaspoons clean water

1 tablespoon rose water
5 drops violet extract

Process : Melt lanolin, petroleum jelly and mineral oil on a medium heat. Heat clean water, rose water and violet-extract in another bowl. Mix the contents of 2 containers and stir till it cools down.

Hand Lotion/Cream

2 tablespoons glycerine
2 tablespoons corn flour (Makki-ka-Ata).
1 cup rose water or orange flower juice

Process: Heat glycerine on a medium heat and gradually add corn flour to it so that the mixture gets thick. Remove this thick mixture from the heat and add rose water or orange flower juice to it. Keep stirring it for about ten minutes.

Skin Tonic

Rose water is the best protector of skin. It was invented by an Arabian doctor in the 10th century. Rose water can be bought at any chemist shop. It can even be prepared at home. Mix 2 tablespoons of rose-essence in four and a half litres of pure clean water. Stir it. Adding a few drops of rose water in your bath water brings freshness.

Cold Cream

4 tablespoons almond oil
1 tablespoon emulsifying wax.
A little scent and a half cucumber.

Process: Peel half a cucumber and cut it into small pieces. Melt almond oil and emulsifying wax on a medium heat and stir it simultaneously. When the two get mixed completely, add cucumber pieces. Now heat the contents for 1 hour on a medium heat. Keep stirring it simultaneously. Then remove resultant thick cream from heat. When it gets cold fill it in a bottle.

You can prepare cold cream from marigold petals also. Take about 50 grams fresh marigold petals, mix it in 2 litres of water taken in a stainless steel pot. Put it on a medium heat, close the lid so that the steam does not escape. Melt emulsifying wax on slow heat in another pot. Now mix the contents of the 2 and heat it for about 15 minutes. Let it get cold. Then fill it in a bottle.

Nourishing Cream

2 tablespoons cocoa butter
2 tablespoons emulsifying wax
1 tablespoon bees-wax
4 tablespoons sesame oil
1 teaspoon almond oil

Process : Put all these ingredients together on medium heat and stir it. When the mixture melts remove it from heat but keep stirring till it gets cold. While it is getting cold, add a few drops of scent. When a thick paste emerges, put it in a bottle.

Eye Cream

1 tablespoon lanolin
1 1/2 tablespoons almond oil
1 teaspoon soyabeen flour
2 teaspoons cold water

Process: Melt lanolin on medium heat. Add almond oil to it. Remove the ensuing thick paste from heat. Add soyabeen powder and cold water to it and stir for 10 minutes. Do not mix any perfume while preparing the eye cream. It might affect the eyes. Using eye-cream is useful if there are circles or dark spots beneath the eyes.

Moisturizer

2 tablespoons bees wax
1 tablespoon liquid wax
5 teaspoons almond oil.
4 teaspoons water
Scent or scented oil (a few drops).

Process: Melt bees-wax and liquid wax in a china bowl. Add amond oil to it. Heat water in another container and then mix it in the first mixture. Remember that both mixtures should be prepared at same temperatures. Stir the thick mixture with a wooden spoon till it gets cold. During the cooling process add scent.

Tooth Powder

Your beauty has no meaning if your teeth are dirty. There is a simple way of preparing tooth powder at home. Mix bicarbonate soda and common salt in 3 : 2 ratio. Brush your teeth regularly with it. Your teeth will look clean and white.

Anti-wrinkle Cream

2 tablespoons lanolin
2 tablespoons almond oil
1 tablespoon apricot oil
3 teaspoons lemon Juice

Process: Mix lanolin, almond oil and apricot oil and heat it on a medium flame. When it melts add lemon juice and perfume. When the mixture becomes a thick paste remove it from the flame and let it get cold. Apricot oil is used as it is full of vitamin 'A'.

Cuticle Cream

3 tablespoons lanolin
2 teaspoons china clay

Process: Mix the two, make it into paste and use it on the nails. There is another simple way of preparing cutical cream. Mix half teaspoon of glycerine in two tablespoons pure petroleum jelly. Use it on nails as cutical cream.

Mouth Wash

1/4 glass vinegar
1/2 glass wine
1 glass honey
1 teaspoon powder of cloves
(tin-pattiya ghas)

Process: Mix all the above together and boil it for 10 minutes. It removes bad breath.

Shampoo

2 eggs
50 gm soapnut (reetha)
50gm dried amla
50 gm shikakai

Process: Grind all the above (except egg) and boil in 2 litres of clean water. Add yolk of 2 eggs to the boiling water. When the mixture gets cold filter it.

Hair Tonic

Many types of hair tonics can be prepared at home for making your hair soft, dense, shining and beautiful. Add 2 tablespoons of henna (*mehandi*) in 2 glasses of boiling water. Wash your hair with it. If you wash your hair with a mixture of 1 tablespoon of vinegar and 2 glasses of water, the roots of your hair will strengthened. Hair become lustrous if you wash it with a mixture of pure water and lemon juice in a ratio of 8 : 1.

Hair Conditioner

1 egg (beaten)
2 tablespoons castor oil
1 teaspoon vinegar
1 teaspoon glycerine

Process: Mix all these together, beat well and massage the roots of your hair with it. It is beneficial to take steam after massage. For making hair conditioner with honey, take 1 egg, add 1 teaspoon of honey and 2 teaspoons of olive oil or coconut oil to it. Mix it thoroughly and use on your hair.

Hair Spray

1 teaspoon pure gum
8 tablespoons water
1 tablespoon alcohol
1/2 teaspoon glycerine

Process: Grind gum and mix with water. Now add alcohol and glycerine to it. Close lid of the bottle and shake it vigorously. Then allow the mixture to remain as such for 24 hours. It will become thick.

Hair-setting Lotion

1 tablespoon castor Oil
1 tablespoon coconut Oil
1 tablespoon vaseline or petroleum jelly
1 teaspoon emulsifying wax
A few drops of scent

Process: Melt all the above on medium heat. Remove it from flame. Add perfume to it and stir. When it gets cold the lotion will be ready for use. If you want to prepare hair cream then you can add 2 teaspoons of lanolin while melting and after removing it from heat add 1 teaspoon of water. Stir the thick mixture till it gets cold.

Vitamin Cream

3 tablespoons lanolin
1/2 tablespoon honey
1 tablespoon soyabean flour or lecithin
4 tablespoons tepid water

Process: Melt lanolin and honey on medium heat and mix it. Now slowly add tepid water to it, keep stirring. Remove it from heat and add soyabeen flour. Keep stirring till it gets cold. Meanwhile you can add scent of your choice.

Vitamins 'E' and 'A' are the ingredients for enhancing beauty. Skin attains a special glow because of these. A cream full of vitamin 'E' can be prepared in the following way:

1 tablespoon bees-wax
1 tablespoon emulsifying wax
1 tablespoon lanolin
3 tablespoons carrot oil (rich in Vit. A)
3 tablespoons wheatgerm oil (rich in Vit. E)
6 teaspoons distilled water
2 drops tincture benzoin
A little orange flower oil.

Process: Melt all these ingredients on medium heat. Now take a separate container and heat water and borax in it till the borax powder is completely dissolved. Now remove both the containers from heat and mix together. Keep stirring till it gets cold. While getting it cold, add a few drops of tincture benzoin. When the thick paste gets cold fill it in a bottle. Sometimes carrot oil and wheatgerm oil is not easily available. In such a case use 5 tablespoons of almond oil, 3 capsules of vitamin E, and 3 vitamin 'A' capsules. These vitamin capsules can be bought from any chemist. Open the capsules and use the powder inside when the paste is getting thick. Stir it thoroughly so that it completely mixes with the cream.

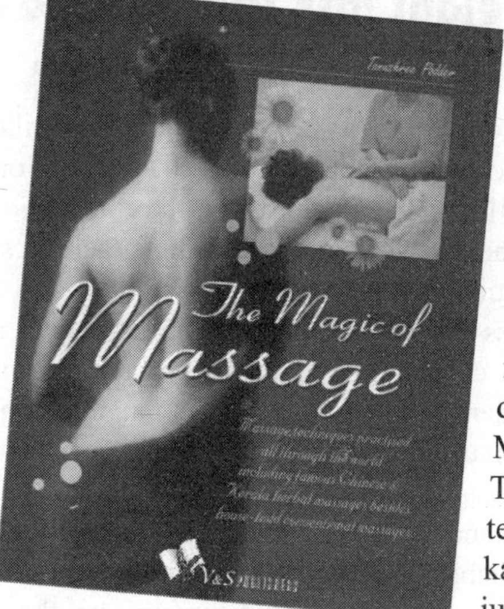

The Magic of Massage

– Tanushree Podder

It is heartening to see how the modern age is rediscovering the beneficial effects of massage.

In fact, right down the ages it has been regarded as one of the most effective therapies for de-stressing. It is unfortunate that the art of massage, which was so intricately woven in our custom is slowly dying a sad death while the western countries have woken up to the Magic of Massage.

This book brings you all the different kinds of massage techniques used all through the world. The Tui Na, Chua-ka, Nuad Bo' Rarn and our famous Kerala Massage are just a few examples of the various types of massage globally popular today.

Big Size • Pages: 173 • • Postage: ₹ 15/-

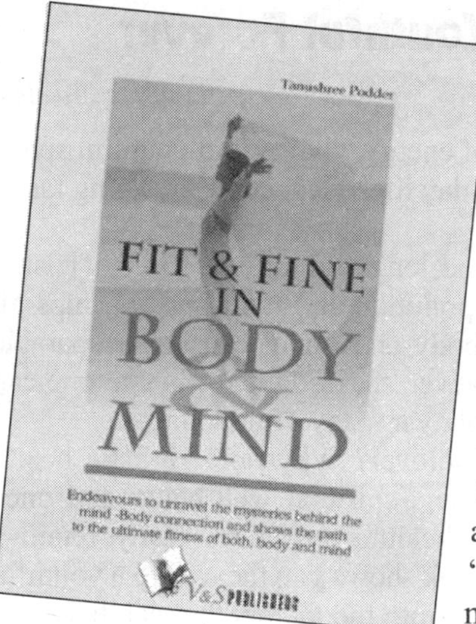

Fit and Fine & Body & Mind

– Tanushree Podder

Hundreds of books are written, every year, on health and fitness but not many reflect on the connection between the mind, body and spirit.

It has been proved beyond doubt that this connection is a vital one and healing of the body cannot take place without the healing of the other two factors. Holistic health is about these three elements. A fitness regime without including all the elements is bound to be ineffective in bringing about 'Total Health Fitness'. This book endeavours to unravel the mysteries behind the mind-body connection and shows the path to the ultimate fitness of both, body and mind.

Demy Size • Pages: 209 • Price: ₹ 108/- • Postage: ₹ 15/-

Ladies weight loss Programme

– Parvesh Handa

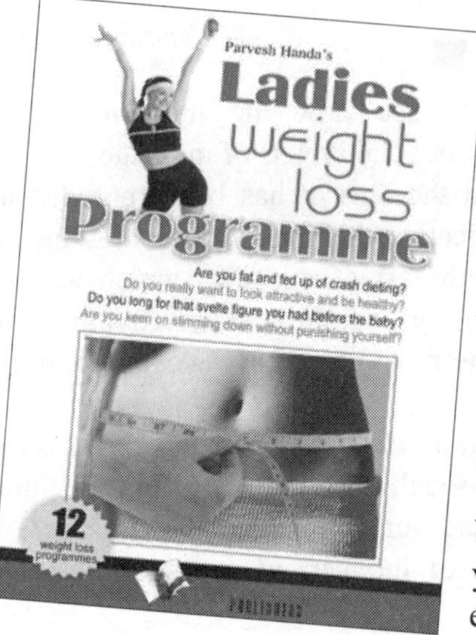

Every woman longs for a beautiful hourglass-like figure. The sight of well-shaped models cat-walking on the ramp allures them. They want to be like them. For this, they go for heavy workouts, crash diets, aerobics, which sometimes click and very often don't.

Ladies Weight Loss Programme aims at understanding a woman's body and covers 12 weight loss programmes. It provides a comprehensive account on topics ranging from cellulite and diet plans to reducing weight to yoga and massage therapies and measures to shed the flab post-pregnancy. It will help you understand the needs and requirements of your body and adopt a suitable simple weight loss programme for yourself. So ladies, no more fretting and fuming over those extra pounds! The perfect figure that you always longed for is just a few pages away.

Demy Size • Pages: 156 • Price: ₹ 95/- • Postage: ₹ 15/-

Stay Youthful Forever

– Tanushree Podder

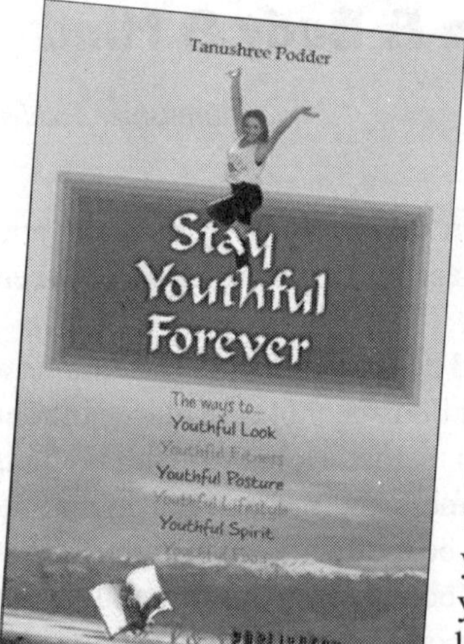

Youth means being full of energy, vitality and youthful spirit. But thanks to the present-day lifestyle, people are aging faster than ever before.

Stress-ridden lives, junk food, long working hours, lack of leisure activities, environmental pollution and toxic relationships all are taking a toll on the body and mind, causing irreparable harm to one's health. However, the good news is that one can have a good enough control over many of these factors.

Can one remain youthful forever? Why not? Holistic health includes physical, mental, and spiritual well-being and once you have attained holistic health, you could easily retain a youthful personality. This book shows you the way to a youthful living— providing an insight into the factors that can help you Stay Youthful Foreever

Demy Size • Pages: 245 • Price: ₹ 120/- • Postage: ₹ 15/-

Housekeeping

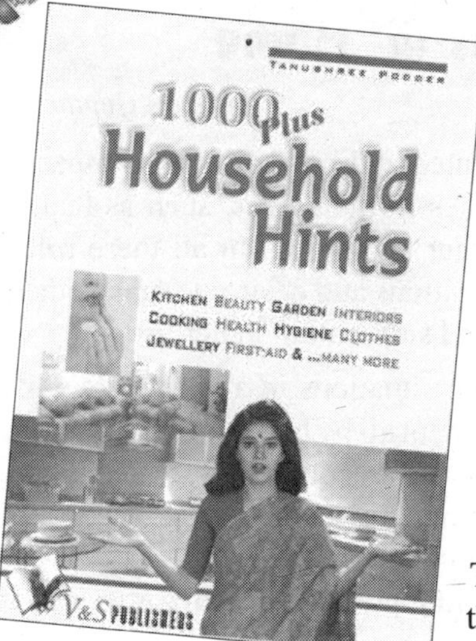

1000 plus Household Hints

– Tanushree Podder

You pride yourself in being a great home-maker.But often you get bogged down by small problems like moss on the kitchen floor, coffee-stains on the shirt, termite on the new wood-work!

This book endeavours to provide easy solutions to common household problems that crop up from time to time. Designed for the young home makers to help them with the running of the household efficiently, it contains more than a 1000 tips on various aspects of home-management.

The wealth of this information is sure to come in handy to the readers.

Demy Size • Pages: 192 • Price: ₹ 150/- • Postage: ₹ 15/-

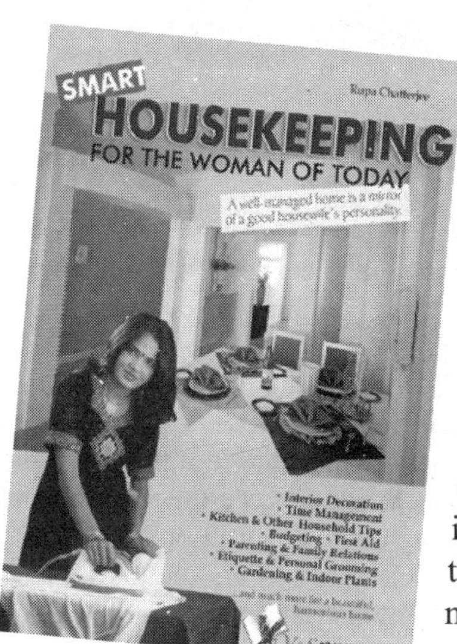

Smart Housekeeping

– Rupa Chatterjee

A beautiful home is the pride and goal of every woman. In fact, a housewife is very often judged by the way she keeps her house. For her it`s like a temple- a key through which she can ensure the highest level of physical and emotional comfort for her family. And in view of its critical significance in one`s life, it`s imperative that your home is managed well .

True, it's an art every homemaker must master. This comprehensive volume written by a seasoned housewife who is also a professional interior designer, is one such handy help that deals with the subject in a critical and comprehensive manner. Never before so many tips and suggestions, covering every aspect of the subject, have been put together in a single volume.

Demy Size • Pages: 292 • Price: ₹ 150/- • Postage: ₹ 15/-

Stress

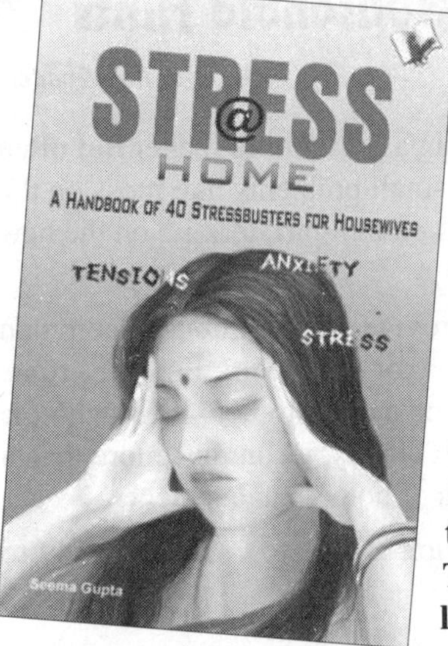

Stress @ Home

– Seema Gupta

Women are naturally talented and have an inborn capacity to play many dynamic roles in their lives, such as that of a daughter, a wife, a mother and so on. In all these roles, she sacrifices her own aspirations and desires to make others happy. This brings stress and suffocation in her life.

The author portrays 40 such situations in a housewife's life telling her how to deal with them all by herself. Certain simple aerobic exercises, morning and evening walks, meditation, listening to good music and reading a book could be some of the stress busters to bring smile on her face.

The book includes tables and charts to measure ones stress levels.

Demy Size • Pages: 183 • Price: ₹ 135/- • Postage: ₹ 15/-

Relationships & Sex

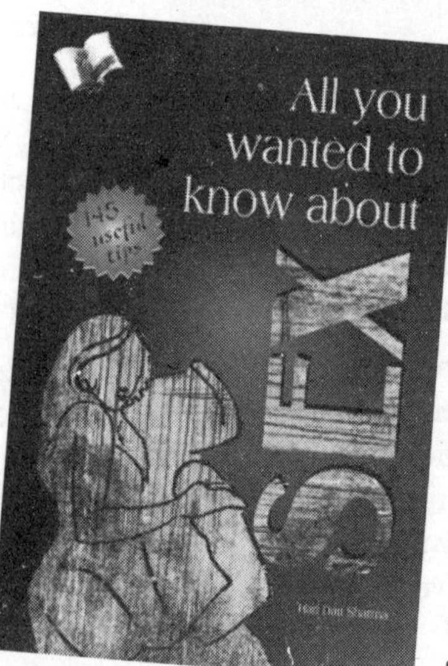

All you wanted to know about Sex

– Rupa Chatterjee

Sex, being a taboo in our society, restricts us from discussing it openly. As a result, several misconceptions and myths are bred and fostered by this denial, leading these myths to gain currency. Will masturbation lead to weakness? Does kissing make you pregnant? Does a wart on the genitalia mean veneral disease?

Unable to find answers to many such queries, these people become easy targets for the quacks who fleece them and in the process give a push to the existing cycle of misinformation.

'All you wanted to know about Sex' throws light on this subject, dispelling scientifically several myths associated with it. The book, from how to enjoy sex, love postures, to techniques of sexual intercourse, discusses threadbare the entire gamut of sexual artistry with references from celebrated sex manuals like Kamasutra and other texts the book contains it all. Backed by apt illustrations, the book will prove to be an informative, educative and enjoyable reading material.

Demy Size • Pages: 144 • Price: ₹ 96/- • Postage: ₹ 15/-

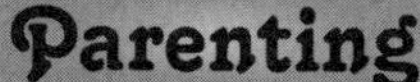

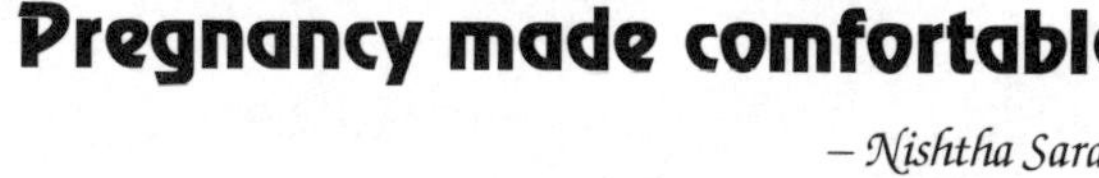

– Nishtha Saraswar

This unique and must read book by Nishtha Saraswat is the only one of its kind that deals with pregnancy related problems with the help of unique combination of yoga and dietetics, two of the most relevant subjects in today`s social context. The effort has been put behind understanding various stages involved in pregnancy in a simple and easy to understand manner. The stress has been laid on providing practical solutions to the common problems faced by women before, during and after pregnancy.

The book has been divided into various sections for ease of reference. The extensive use of pictures, tables, illustrations and testimonials lends practicality to the book and makes it user-friendly. The book aims at becoming a complete reference manual during the journey from planning pregnancy to getting back in a healthy shape post pregnancy. Aspiring mothers will f nd this book indispensable in their daily lives. Regular reference and usage of the book during pregnancy will ensure that pregnancy becomes a comfortable and pleasant experience for all women.

Demy Size • Pages: 129 • Price: ₹ 150/- • Postage: ₹ 15/-

Raising a Daughter in 21st Century India

– Rupa Chatterjee

Every environment makes its own specif c social and moral demands on the individual. As such, in the Indian environment today raising a daughter is not what it used to be a few decades earlier. Keeping this in view, the book has been created especially for the mothers of today. The mother of two daughters, the author has used both her own experiences and suggestions from peers to give valuable insights on bringing up a daughter in 21st century India.

She has not only attempted to highlight the problems of bringing up a daughter today, but also tried to show how these can be tackled, blending our traditional values to bring up a well-adjusted daughter. The book contains time-tested tips, practical suggestions and reliable recommendations, with insights from pediatricians, psychiatrists, teachers and other experts, and will serve as an effective guide for all mothers, particularly f rst-time mothers. Peppered with numerous f rst-person accounts, the book can serve as a handy guide in moments of trying tension, while dealing with your teenage daughter.

Demy Size • Pages: 136 • Price: ₹ 120/- • Postage: ₹ 15/-